PREM

A DARK LOVE STORY

Author's Note

Prem was originally written as an original feature film screenplay with a cinematic structure and visual rhythm. This novel is an adaptation of that screenplay, created to let readers experience the story beyond the screen.

The work is imaginative in nature and shaped by subconscious thought and psychological observation. Portions of the adaptation process were assisted by artificial intelligence as a creative tool.

Thank you for reading.

— Nanda

Characters

Prem

A highly successful criminal advocate whose brilliance lies not only in the courtroom but in control itself. Calculated, obsessive, and meticulously ordered, Prem believes rare things must be preserved, not exposed. His love is not impulsive but architectural, built patiently over years. He designs environments, routines, and people with the same precision, and once something belongs to him, he ensures it never escapes. To the world, he is respected. Within the estate, he is absolute.

Madhu

An English literature graduate, gentle, observant, and uniquely beautiful from her school days. Drawn to freedom, birds, and open skies in her earlier life, Madhu gradually loses her sense of self without ever realizing it. Her journey is not marked by resistance or rebellion, but by quiet acceptance. She never learns the truth about what is taken from her, and that ignorance becomes the most devastating part of her fate.

Arjun

A software engineer from another part of Karnataka, practical, sincere, and emotionally straightforward. Arjun represents a life Madhu could have lived, ordinary but free. His engagement to Madhu triggers Prem's final descent into irreversible action. His death is presented to the world as an accident, and his truth is buried before it can speak.

Prem's Mother

An educated woman and homemaker who understands her son's nature better than anyone else. She recognizes Prem's obsession and control from his childhood, though she never imagines it would reach its darkest form. When she finally realizes the truth behind Arjun's death, her knowledge becomes dangerous. Her death ensures Prem's obsession succeeds, while also granting him the sympathy of being motherless.

Prem's Father
A renowned criminal lawyer whose success and moral flexibility shape Prem's worldview. His wealth and reputation provide the foundation upon which Prem builds his life, education, and influence. Though largely absent in the later narrative, his legacy permeates Prem's beliefs about power, law, and consequence.

Madhu's Father
A bank employee, disciplined and principled, representing stability and middle-class values. He loves his daughter deeply but fails to perceive the silent transformation taking place within her life.

Madhu's Mother
A homemaker, emotionally intuitive yet restrained by trust in social structures. She senses change in Madhu but interprets it as healing and comfort rather than confinement.

Ujju Baba
A shadowy facilitator who assists Prem in matters that must remain outside legality. He represents the unseen mechanisms that allow Prem's plans to succeed without leaving visible stains.

The Estate Servants
Quiet, obedient, and selectively blind. They move within the estate without questioning its design or the lives unfolding inside it. Their silence sustains the system as effectively as Prem's control.

The Estate
More than a setting, the estate functions as a living system. With its gardens, deer enclosure, bird cages, swimming pool, tennis court, and glass house, it embodies Prem's philosophy of preservation through limitation. Over time, it becomes Madhu's entire world, absorbing her identity until the boundary between place and person disappears.

EVERY LOVE STORY HAS A TRUTH; NOT EVERY TRUTH ARRIVES IN TIME

Chapter One
The Colony and the Watching

The colony woke before the sun fully cleared the rooftops.

Water swept across cement verandas in long practiced arcs. Buckets clanged softly. A radio hummed from somewhere down the lane, the voice low, almost apologetic, as if it knew the day had not yet agreed to begin. The air carried the smell of wet dust and milk boiling over. Gates opened one by one, each with its own sound, some sharp, some tired, some recently oiled.

The houses stood close together, shoulder to shoulder, sharing walls and habits. Paint peeled in places where years had won small battles. Windows remained open. Lives here did not hide. Children moved through the mornings in uniforms that marked difference more clearly than names ever could.

Prem stood on the balcony of his house and watched.

He was thirteen, tall for his age, quiet in a way that did not invite questions. His school bag rested near the door behind him, zipped, books aligned. His shoes were clean, placed side by side, laces tucked in neatly. Everything around him was prepared. There was no rush in him, no uncertainty about what came next.

From the balcony, he could see most of the colony road. The turn near the temple. The narrow stretch where scooters squeezed past each other without apology. The small park at the far end with a slide that no longer shone and swings that complained when pushed too hard.

He was waiting for a particular moment.

Below, a gate opened.

Madhu stepped out of her house with her school bag hanging low on her back. Her hair was braided tightly, the braid ending just below her shoulders, tied with black ribbons that caught the light when she moved. Her uniform was clean but worn at the edges, fabric softened by repeated washing. Her socks were pulled up carefully, though one had already begun to slip.

Her mother followed her to the gate, fingers quick as they adjusted the bag strap, smoothing the braid once more. Her father stood nearby with his helmet in one hand and a steel lunch box in the other. He spoke briefly, his voice calm, practical. Madhu listened, nodding, serious in a way children sometimes are when they understand responsibility but not yet its weight.

She bent down to touch her mother's feet, then her father's. They smiled at her, proud and unguarded.

Prem did not move.

Madhu climbed onto the back of her father's bike. The engine started with a low cough. She held the side bar lightly, posture straight, eyes forward. As the bike moved, wind lifted loose strands of her hair, freeing them briefly from the braid before they settled again.

The bike passed through the colony road slowly, weaving around puddles and people. Madhu did not look around. She did not look up. She did not know she was being watched.

Prem leaned slightly forward, his hands resting on the balcony railing.

Every morning, this scene repeated itself with minor variations. Sometimes the bike moved faster. Sometimes slower. Sometimes her mother lingered longer at the gate. Sometimes her father said something that made her laugh briefly before the helmet hid her face.

Prem noticed all of it.

He noticed how the bike exposed her to the road. How close other vehicles passed. How she moved through space without protection, without glass, without barriers. He noticed the way people looked at her, briefly, without knowing why.

He noticed, and he remembered.

When the bike turned the corner and disappeared from view, Prem straightened. He picked up his bag and walked inside.

The difference between outside and inside was immediate.

The colony sounds dulled the moment the door closed. The house absorbed noise differently. The walls were thicker. The rooms larger. The silence more intentional. Curtains filtered the light so it entered without revealing too much.

His mother stood near the dining table, placing a glass of milk beside his plate. She was educated, careful with her words, precise in her movements. She had chosen to stay home, and she managed the house with the same attention others gave to careers.

"You are early," she said.

"I woke up early," Prem replied.

She looked at him closely, as she often did. Not searching for faults, but for alignment. "Did you sleep well"

"Yes."

That was enough.

His father entered moments later, already dressed for court, his presence filling the room without effort. He was a successful criminal lawyer, known well beyond the colony. His name carried weight. His voice carried certainty.

"Ready" his father asked.

"Yes," Prem said.

They ate quickly. Conversation stayed practical. His father commented briefly on a case, on how people misunderstood evidence, on how truth was rarely what mattered in a courtroom. Prem listened without interruption. He did not ask questions. He absorbed tone, not instruction.

Outside, the car waited.

The driver opened the door. Prem got in and sat quietly in the back seat. As the car moved through the colony gate, Prem looked out once more at the road Madhu had taken. It was empty now, swept clean, ordinary again.

School passed as it always did.

Prem excelled without drama. Teachers praised him. Classmates respected him from a distance. He did not seek friendships. He did not feel their absence. His mind moved in patterns that did not require company.

In the afternoons, the car brought him back.

He timed his return unconsciously. Homework was completed quickly, accurately. His mother checked his work, corrected a minor error, nodded in approval. She liked order. So did he.

Later, as the sun softened and shadows stretched across the road, Madhu returned.

Sometimes she walked with friends, their voices low, their laughter contained. Sometimes she walked alone, her pace slower now, her shoulders relaxed. Her braid loosened over time. Eventually, it disappeared, replaced by a simple ponytail.

Prem watched from different places. The balcony. The window. The staircase where a curtain partially hid him. He did not always choose the same spot. He preferred variation in vantage, not in routine.

Years passed.

The colony changed in small ways. New paint. New tenants. Old faces replaced. Madhu grew taller. Her features sharpened. Her beauty, already present, became unmistakable. It drew attention without effort. Teachers noticed. Neighbors commented. Boys looked.

Prem watched them look.

He noted which ones stared too long. Which ones tried to speak. Which ones followed her with their eyes as she passed. He remembered faces. Names when he learned them. He did not interfere. Not yet.

His own life expanded outward.

He left the colony for higher studies. Lived in hostels where noise never fully slept. Returned during holidays, then for good. His father's legacy opened doors. He learned the law not as justice, but as structure. As a way to decide outcomes.

Still, he asked about the colony.

Casually. Indirectly.

"How is everyone" he would ask his mother.

She would mention weddings, transfers, illnesses. Sometimes, she would say Madhu's name.

"She is doing well," she would say. "Studying hard. Very bright."

Prem stored that information.

When he returned permanently, the colony felt smaller.

Madhu was no longer a schoolgirl. She taught now. She walked differently. Carried herself with quiet confidence. She still did not look up at his house. She still did not know him beyond reputation.

That did not trouble him.

Watching had never required acknowledgment.

One evening, as Prem stood by the window, a bird flew across the colony road. A small thing, quick and unremarkable, cutting through the open space between houses before vanishing beyond the trees.

Madhu paused briefly to watch it.

Prem noticed the pause.

He followed the bird's path with his eyes until it disappeared.

Then he looked back at Madhu, already walking again.

Waiting had never felt like waiting to him.

It felt like ownership taking its time.

Chapter Two
Patterns and Inheritance

The first thing Prem learned was that order did not announce itself.

It revealed itself slowly, through repetition. Through the comfort of predictability. Through the absence of surprise.

His house taught him this before his father ever did.

Doors were closed at specific hours. Lights were dimmed rather than switched off abruptly. Shoes were placed with their toes aligned. Newspapers were folded, not left open. Even arguments, when they happened, ended before voices rose.

Prem absorbed these rules without being told. He understood early that disorder was not punished loudly. It was corrected quietly.

His mother watched him closely as he grew.

She noticed how he arranged his toys as a child, not in piles but in lines. How he grew irritated when something was moved without reason. How he remembered exactly where he had placed something days earlier and reacted with visible discomfort when it was not there.

She did not scold him.

She adjusted the environment instead.

She kept his room consistent. She warned servants not to rearrange his things. She explained changes before making them. She believed structure would soothe him.

It did.

Prem did not throw tantrums. He did not rebel. He complied completely when rules aligned with his sense of order. When they did not, he withdrew into silence.

Silence was his way of control.

His father recognized this differently.

He saw discipline. Focus. Potential.

He took Prem with him occasionally, not to courtrooms at first, but to chambers. To offices where files moved faster than people. Where men spoke softly about things that destroyed lives.

Prem sat quietly in a corner, reading or pretending to, while his father spoke to clients. He listened without appearing to. He learned how desperation sounded. How lies softened when fear rose. How confidence could be manufactured through tone alone.

On the drive back, his father sometimes spoke.

"People think the law is about truth," he would say. "It is not. It is about convincing others which truth to accept."

Prem listened. He did not ask questions.

He did not need to.

At home, his mother noticed the change in him after these visits. Not excitement. Not confusion. Something steadier.

He began to ask for fewer things. But when he asked, he expected precision. He wanted answers that fit exactly. Explanations that closed all gaps.

He did not like maybe.

He did not like later.

He did not like chance.

In the colony, Madhu continued to exist just beyond his reach.

She changed schools. Her uniform changed color. Her bag changed shape. Her beauty sharpened into something that drew longer looks now. Prem noticed the way people's heads turned when she passed, the way attention followed her without invitation.

He felt something tighten inside him when that happened.

Not jealousy.

Unease.

He watched her father's bike more closely now. The way it navigated traffic. The way other vehicles passed too near. The way her presence drew attention she did not manage.

Once, a car slowed beside the bike. The driver looked too long. Madhu shifted slightly, uncomfortable. Her father did not notice.

Prem noticed.

The car moved on. Nothing happened.

But something settled in Prem then, quietly.

He understood that beauty was exposure.

Exposure required management.

That evening, Prem sat at the dining table longer than usual, his food untouched.

His mother watched him.

"What are you thinking" she asked.

"Nothing," Prem replied.

She waited. She knew when he was withholding.

After a moment, he said, "Why do people stare"

"At what"

"At things that are not theirs."

She did not answer immediately. "Some people do not know how to look properly."

He considered this. "They spoil things."

She looked at him sharply then, a flicker of concern passing across her face. "People do not spoil things just by looking."

"Sometimes they do," Prem said.

She chose her response carefully. "That is why some things need protection. But protection should not become imprisonment."

He nodded. But he did not fully accept it.

Protection, to him, meant limits.

Limits meant safety.

As he grew older, his patterns intensified.

He chose his friends carefully. Few. Predictable. People who did not surprise him. When someone behaved unexpectedly, he distanced himself without explanation.

At school, teachers admired his focus. He did not argue. He did not disrupt. He delivered exactly what was expected, and often more.

At home, servants learned quickly how to move around him. Not because he demanded it aloud, but because deviation made him still. Silence from Prem was not peace. It was warning.

His mother understood this language.

She intervened when necessary, softened edges where she could. She reminded him to smile when required. To speak kindly even when he felt detached. She worried quietly, never openly.

She believed his rigidity would mellow with age.

She had seen boys with strong patterns loosen as they grew.

She had not seen Prem loosen at all.

When Prem began driving, his father offered him a driver immediately.

Prem refused.

"I'll drive myself," he said.

"It's not safe," his mother said. "You can think better if someone else drives."

"I think better when I drive," Prem replied.

He disliked the presence of a driver. Too much observation. Too many variables. Another person meant another witness to timing, destinations, pauses.

Driving became his private space.

He chose his routes carefully. Preferred roads with predictable flow. Avoided areas where randomness ruled. He did not honk unnecessarily. He did not speed for thrill.

He drove to arrive, not to experience movement.

When he later began his practice, he replicated this philosophy everywhere.

His office had two junior advocates. No more. No less.

He selected them carefully. Intelligent, but not ambitious enough to challenge. Loyal to structure. Comfortable executing instructions without seeking authorship.

Two clerks handled paperwork. Both precise. Both habitual. Both trained to follow pattern rather than initiative.

He did not believe in large teams.

Large teams created noise.

Noise created error.

He drove himself to work most days. Rarely, if circumstances forced him to use a driver, he chose someone recommended for silence rather than skill. The arrangement never lasted long.

At the center of his office sat the typewriter.

An old machine, restored and maintained personally by Prem. He had several. Each serviced regularly. Each kept clean, oiled, precise.

He drafted everything on them.

Legal arguments. Notes. Letters.

No computer.

No digital drafts.

Each key press was deliberate. Audible. Final.

The sound filled the office at night when others had left. It filled the house when he worked late. It filled the estate later, becoming a rhythm others learned to live around.

Madhu heard that sound for the first time years later and thought it comforting.

Prem's mother had heard it much earlier.

She knew that sound meant resolution.

She had learned to listen for changes in its rhythm. Faster meant agitation. Slower meant certainty.

As Prem's career flourished, the colony spoke of him with pride.

The lawyer's son. Now a successful advocate himself. Sharp. Reliable. Powerful.

Madhu knew his name well by then.

She knew him as reputation. As distance. As someone from a world that did not overlap with hers.

She did not know the boy who had watched her from balconies and car windows.

She did not know the man who believed rare things needed limits.

And Prem did not hurry to bridge that gap.

He had never rushed anything that mattered.

Some patterns, he believed, deserved time.

Chapter Three
The Estate

The estate did not announce itself.

It did not rise suddenly or impose itself on the road. It revealed itself slowly, through distance. First the boundary wall appeared, longer than expected, unbroken, pale against the dust. Then the gate, wide and heavy, opening without sound. Beyond it, a stretch of driveway that bent slightly, refusing a direct line of sight to what lay inside.

Prem preferred it that way.

He had inherited the land before he had inherited the house. His father had believed in visibility. Big gates. Straight paths. A sense of arrival. Prem redesigned everything after his father's death. Curves replaced lines. Trees replaced openness. Silence replaced display.

The estate became a space that did not invite inspection.

Inside, the air changed.

The city noise fell away as if absorbed by the ground itself. Even birds sounded different here, their calls softer, contained. The garden unfolded gradually, lawns cut precisely, hedges trimmed to their limits, paths edged with stone. Nothing spilled. Nothing grew wild.

Prem walked through it in the early mornings, his steps measured, his attention divided between the path ahead and the details that confirmed continuity. A leaf out of place. A stone slightly shifted. A branch that had grown faster than expected.

These were not irritations. They were signals.

The gardeners learned quickly.

They arrived early, worked silently, and left without commentary. Instructions were followed exactly. Questions were discouraged not by reprimand, but by the quiet certainty that they were unnecessary.

The servants lived on the edge of the estate, their quarters modest, separate, contained. They moved through the house with an understanding that had never been spoken aloud. Doors were opened before they were needed. Food appeared without being requested. Rooms were cleaned while still feeling undisturbed.

Obedience here was not enforced.

It was cultivated.

Prem liked it that way.

The swimming pool lay beyond the garden, a long rectangle of water that reflected the sky without distortion. It was cleaned daily. The water level maintained precisely. No leaves floated on its surface. No ripples disturbed it unless someone chose to enter.

Prem rarely swam.

The pool was not for recreation. It was for completeness. A space that suggested possibility without demanding use.

Beyond it lay the tennis court.

The surface was pristine. The net taut. The lines repainted regularly. No shoes marked it. No rackets lay forgotten at its edge. It existed as proof of discipline rather than play.

Further still, a small playground stood.

Slides. Swings. A climbing frame.

They were rarely used.

Prem had not removed them because absence would raise questions. He preferred presence without activity. It reminded him that not everything had to be consumed to be controlled.

At the far edge of the estate, partially hidden by trees, stood the aviary.

Madhu noticed it the first time she visited.

She had arrived late that evening, exhausted, numb, carrying nothing but a bag and the weight of days that refused to organize themselves. The house had absorbed her quietly, offering space without demand. Prem's mother had guided her gently, without questions, without explanations.

In the morning, Madhu stepped outside.

The garden surprised her. Not its size, but its restraint. Nothing shouted. Nothing competed. The space felt watched rather than lived in.

She walked slowly, following the path until she heard the sound.

Birds.

She stopped.

The aviary stood behind a screen of foliage, large enough to house dozens of birds. Some perched quietly. Others moved restlessly within their limits. Colors flashed. Wings spread and folded. Song rose and fell in careful rhythms.

Madhu approached, her steps hesitant.

"They are beautiful," she said.

Prem stood a little behind her. "They are rare."

She turned. "Are they"

"Yes."

She watched them closely now. Their feathers gleamed. Their eyes were alert. They looked healthy, well fed.

“They are not free,” she said.

Prem did not respond immediately.

“Freedom is overrated,” he said finally. “Especially for rare things.”

She frowned slightly. “I like seeing birds fly.”

“You can still see them fly,” he replied, gesturing to the space within the aviary. “Just not disappear.”

She studied his face, trying to understand whether he was joking. He was not.

“Out there,” she said, pointing upward, “they choose where to go.”

“They also get hunted,” Prem said. “They get injured. They die unnoticed.”

She looked back at the birds.

“They look safe,” she admitted.

“They are preserved,” Prem said. “The world is careless with beauty. People spoil what they admire. I don’t trust chance with rare things.”

Madhu said nothing more. She did not argue. The birds sang softly, unconcerned.

Later, she would think about that conversation without discomfort.

At the time, it felt reasonable.

Prem returned to his routines quickly after she arrived.

His office remained unchanged.

Two juniors arrived before him every morning, reviewing files quietly, organizing notes, preparing arguments without speculation. Two clerks handled paperwork with mechanical precision, their movements habitual, their presence unobtrusive.

Prem arrived on time, every day.

He drove himself.

The car was an extension of his office. Clean. Silent. Predictable. He did not play music. He did not take calls unless necessary. Driving was a space for thinking, not interruption.

In the evenings, he returned to the estate and worked late.

The typing machine waited in his study, polished, maintained, reliable. He preferred the weight of the keys, the resistance before each letter appeared. The sound anchored him. It forced intention. Each sentence existed because he had committed to it physically.

Madhu heard the typing at night.

At first, it unsettled her. Then it comforted her. The sound suggested certainty. Someone awake. Someone handling things.

Prem's mother heard it too.

She had heard it for years.

She knew the difference between agitation and resolve by its rhythm. She noticed how, after Madhu arrived, the typing slowed. Evened out. It carried a steadiness that suggested something had settled.

She did not comment.

She watched Madhu move through the estate, curious but cautious. She noticed how the servants responded to her, gentle but precise. How meals adjusted to her preferences without being asked. How paths seemed to align to her movements.

She recognized the pattern.

Prem had done this before.

With objects. With routines. With space.

Never with a person.

The estate adjusted itself around Madhu quietly.

Her room was changed slightly after the first week. Curtains replaced. A chair added near the window. Books appeared on the shelf, titles chosen carefully, familiar enough to be comforting, unfamiliar enough to suggest growth.

Madhu noticed, but did not question.

She spent afternoons in the garden, reading, watching birds at the edge of the estate fly freely above the boundary wall. She smiled when they crossed the sky without restriction.

Prem noticed where she stood when she watched them.

He adjusted the schedule of the gardeners so that path remained clear at that hour.

In the evenings, Madhu sometimes walked near the aviary again.

The birds recognized her presence quickly. They moved closer. Some sang louder. She spoke to them softly, telling them nothing important.

Prem watched from a distance.

He believed the birds sensed intention.

At the office, Prem won cases.

Not loudly. Not theatrically.

He dismantled narratives patiently. He questioned witnesses without aggression. He let pauses do the work words could not. Judges listened. Opposing counsel hesitated.

Clients trusted him without understanding why.

When asked how he managed outcomes others could not, Prem replied simply, "I prepare."

Preparation, to him, was not effort.

It was alignment.

One afternoon, a junior asked him why he insisted on drafting arguments on the old machine when computers were faster.

Prem looked at him briefly.

"Speed creates noise," he said. "Noise creates error."

The junior nodded and did not ask again.

That night, Madhu sat by the pool, feet near the edge, watching the water reflect the sky. It was still. Perfectly still.

"I used to swim in rivers when I was a child," she said when Prem joined her. "The water never stayed like this."

"It's easier to maintain when it's contained," Prem replied.

She smiled faintly. "You like control."

"I like responsibility," he said.

She accepted the answer.

The estate settled into its rhythm.

Days passed without urgency. Nights arrived without disruption. The garden grew. The pool remained unused. The tennis court stayed pristine. The birds sang.

Madhu felt safe.

Prem felt complete.

And somewhere beyond the boundary wall, birds continued to fly freely, unseen, unheard, irrelevant.

The estate did not notice them.

Neither did Prem.

Among the trees stood a glass structure that caught light differently, reflective and unreadable, dismissed by Madhu as another indulgence of the estate.

Beyond the trimmed lawns, fenced greenery moved quietly, something living and contained, though Madhu did not stop to look.

Chapter Four
Convergence

Madhu met Arjun without ceremony.

There was no dramatic introduction, no moment she would later identify as the beginning. It happened the way most real connections do, through people who already knew each other, through conversations that were not meant to matter.

A friend invited her for coffee after class. Another friend joined. Arjun arrived late, apologetic, helmet in hand, laptop bag slung over his shoulder. He smiled easily, the kind of smile that did not demand attention but held it anyway.

They spoke about nothing important at first.

Work. Traffic. A mutual irritation with how loud cafés had become. Madhu noticed that he listened when she spoke, not waiting for his turn. Arjun noticed that she chose her words carefully, as if they mattered even when the topic did not.

When they parted, neither of them thought of it as a meeting.

They met again because there was no reason not to.

The group grew smaller over time. Friends dropped away naturally, schedules misaligned, priorities shifted. Eventually, it was just the two of them sitting across from each other, talking longer than necessary, leaving later than planned.

Madhu liked that Arjun did not interrupt her silences.

He worked as a software engineer, B.Tech degree from another part of Karnataka, his family rooted far from Bangalore. He spoke of his work plainly, without glamour. Systems. Deadlines. Problems solved quietly. He liked clarity. He liked things that worked.

She spoke of literature, of how stories revealed people more honestly than conversations did. He listened without pretending to understand everything.

They balanced each other without effort.

Madhu's parents noticed the change before she did.

She smiled more often. Stayed out later. Checked her phone absentmindedly while helping her mother in the kitchen. Her father watched quietly, observant in the way men who work with numbers often are.

"Who is he," her mother asked one evening, not accusing, simply curious.

"A friend," Madhu said.

Her mother smiled. "Friends don't usually make people forget to eat."

Madhu laughed and did not answer.

When she told them about Arjun properly, there was no resistance.

A software engineer. Good education. Steady job. From a respectable family. Not from their colony, not from Prem's world, but solid, understandable.

Her father approved quietly. Her mother asked practical questions. Madhu answered them all honestly.

She did not mention Prem.

There was no reason to.

Arjun proposed on an ordinary evening.

They were sitting in his car, parked near a stretch of road that overlooked the city lights. Traffic moved below them, constant, unremarkable. He spoke without rehearsal, his voice steady, his words simple.

"I don't want to wait too long," he said. "I know what I want."

Madhu did not answer immediately.

She looked out at the city, the lights blurring slightly. She thought of her parents. Of her work. Of the life she had imagined vaguely but never detailed.

She thought of how calm she felt with him.

"Yes," she said finally.

Arjun exhaled slowly, relief breaking through his composure. He smiled, reached for her hand, then stopped, waiting.

She placed her hand in his.

They decided on an engagement first. Time to inform families. Time to plan properly. No rush, but no uncertainty either.

Madhu told her parents the next day.

Her mother cried softly, already thinking ahead. Her father nodded, practical, satisfied.

The news traveled quickly through their circle.

And then it reached the colony.

Prem heard about it in passing.

A conversation he was not meant to listen to. A name mentioned casually. Madhu's name, followed by engagement, followed by congratulations.

He did not react immediately.

He finished the document he was drafting, his fingers steady on the keys of the typewriter. The sound remained even, controlled.

Only when he reached the end of the page did he pause.

The silence that followed felt heavier than sound.

That evening, Prem drove longer than usual.

He chose routes that circled back on themselves, roads that allowed uninterrupted movement. He did not turn on the radio. He did not call anyone.

He thought.

The engagement changed everything.

Before, Madhu's life had been in motion, but motion could be redirected. Choices could be reconsidered. Time existed as space.

An engagement closed doors.

It made her future visible to others.

It made her unavailable.

That night, Prem did not sleep.

He sat in his study, the typewriter untouched, his hands resting on the desk. His thoughts did not race. They aligned.

By morning, he had reached a conclusion.

He did not express it aloud.

At breakfast, his mother noticed the shift.

Not agitation. Not anger.

A narrowing.

"You look tired," she said.

"I'm fine," Prem replied.

She studied him longer than usual. "Is something bothering you"

"No," he said. "Something has clarified."

She did not like the word.

At the office, Prem worked with renewed focus.

He reviewed Arjun's name once more, now intentionally. The file was thin. Ordinary. No significance on its own. A man moving through systems without friction.

Prem learned his routes without effort. Workplaces revealed themselves through patterns. Timing repeated. Behavior stabilized.

This was not obsession taking shape.

It was obsession stepping forward.

Meanwhile, Madhu moved through her days unaware of the shift.

She told Arjun about Prem only in passing.

"He's from my colony," she said. "A big advocate now. Very respected."

Arjun nodded. "Sounds important."

"He's helpful," she added, thinking of how smoothly things had gone lately, of how some administrative issues at work had resolved unexpectedly.

She did not connect the dots.

At the estate, the birds sang.

Prem walked past the aviary one evening and stopped briefly. A bird fluttered against the edge of its space, then settled.

He watched it calmly.

Rare things needed protection.

He had believed that since he was a boy.

That night, the typewriter came alive again.

The sound was slow. Deliberate. Each key press carried weight.

Prem's mother listened from her room, her hands folded in her lap. She recognized the rhythm.

Not urgency.

Decision.

Outside the estate walls, Madhu and Arjun spoke about venues and dates, about how quickly time seemed to be moving now that it had shape.

Madhu felt hopeful.

She felt chosen.

She did not know that someone else had already decided the shape of her future.

And Prem did not doubt himself.

He never had.

Chapter Five
Preparation without Urgency

Prem did not hurry.

Haste, he believed, introduced error. Error invited attention. Attention created questions. Questions were the enemy of completion.

The engagement announcement did not alter his routines outwardly. He woke at the same hour. He drove the same roads. He entered his office with the same measured nod to the receptionist, the same brief glance at the day's schedule, the same expectation that everything would be where it belonged.

But inside him, something had aligned.

He began to notice the city differently. Not as movement, but as sequence. Signals. Interruptions. Places where certainty thinned and chance pretended to rule. He did not seek danger. He sought indifference. Places where nothing mattered long enough to be remembered.

At the office, the two juniors worked quietly at their desks. Files were sorted. Notes prepared. One of them asked a question about a witness statement in a pending case.

Prem listened, then answered with three sentences. Precise. Final. The junior nodded and returned to his work.

Prem did not raise his voice. He never needed to.

The clerks moved paper from one place to another, stamping, filing, aligning. They knew which documents required his signature and which did not. They knew which files he wanted on his desk before he asked for them.

This was not loyalty. It was conditioning.

During lunch, Prem did not eat with his colleagues. He preferred the quiet of his office. He ate lightly, wiped his hands carefully, then turned to the typewriter.

The machine waited.

He rolled in a fresh sheet, adjusted the margin, tested a key once. The sound echoed briefly, sharp and contained.

He began drafting.

Not about Arjun. Not yet.

He worked on a case involving a fatal incident. A construction site. A man who had fallen. Responsibility blurred between contractor and circumstance. Prem shaped the argument carefully, allowing the narrative to settle where it would cause the least friction.

When he finished, he leaned back and closed his eyes for a moment.

He was not practicing.

He was aligning.

That evening, Prem drove past Madhu's street without stopping. He did not slow the car. He did not look toward her house. He already knew where she would be, what time she would return, who she would be with.

Observation was useful only when it revealed something new.

At the estate, the garden was being watered. The gardeners moved in straight lines, hoses angled precisely. Prem walked the path that ran along the edge of the lawn, his shoes leaving no imprint.

He stopped at the aviary.

The birds stirred as he approached, wings fluttering briefly before settling again. He watched them closely, noting the way they adapted to boundaries. They did not fight the enclosure. They learned it.

His mother watched him from a distance.

She had seen this look before. Not often. It appeared when Prem reached conclusions that did not invite discussion.

She waited until dinner.

"You've been quiet," she said, serving the food.

"I've been thinking," Prem replied.

She nodded. "About work"

"About arrangements."

She paused, her hand hovering briefly over the serving spoon. "Arrangements for what"

"For things that will change," he said.

She sat down slowly. "Things always change."

"Yes," Prem agreed. "But not without direction."

She studied him carefully. "Madhu's engagement," she said, not accusing, not probing. Naming the obvious.

"Yes."

Her expression softened, relief passing through her features. "That's good. She deserves happiness."

Prem did not respond immediately. He ate a few bites, placed his cutlery down carefully.

"Happiness is fragile," he said. "It needs protection."

His mother felt a familiar tightening in her chest. She had heard this logic before, in different forms, across many years.

"Protection should not become interference," she said gently.

He looked at her then, really looked. "Everything that lasts is interfered with."

She did not argue. She had learned when silence was safer.

In the days that followed, Prem's attention moved outward, away from the estate and into the city. He did not follow Arjun directly. He did not trail him or watch him obsessively.

He allowed information to come to him.

People spoke easily around Prem. They mistook his quiet for disinterest. They filled it with details.

A clerk mentioned a traffic delay near a particular junction. A junior complained about road work that had dragged on for months. A client spoke of a minor accident he had witnessed, shrugged it off as inevitable.

Prem stored these details without reaction.

He drove those roads himself, at different times of day. Morning. Evening. Late night. He observed how vehicles behaved when lanes narrowed, how patience dissolved when signals lagged, how people made assumptions when rules blurred.

He did not take notes.

He remembered.

At home, Madhu moved through her days buoyed by plans. She spoke with Arjun about venues, about dates that worked for both families, about practicalities that made the future feel real.

She mentioned Prem occasionally, always positively.

"He helped me with some paperwork at work," she told Arjun one evening. "He knows everyone. Things get done when he's involved."

Arjun smiled. "Sounds like a useful person to know."

"Yes," Madhu agreed. "He's very composed."

Arjun did not think about Prem again.

Why would he.

At the estate, Prem's mother began to notice small changes.

Prem returned later some nights, his car headlights cutting across the driveway long after dinner had ended. He ate alone, quietly, then went to his study. The typewriter sounded different now.

Not faster.

More deliberate.

Each key press arrived with equal weight, like steps placed carefully on unfamiliar ground.

She listened from her room, counting nothing, measuring nothing, only absorbing rhythm. She could not have said why it unsettled her.

One afternoon, she walked into the study unannounced.

Prem sat at the desk, the machine idle, a sheet half-filled. He looked up calmly.

"Do you need something" he asked.

She shook her head. "I just wanted to see you."

Her gaze drifted to the typewriter, to the neat lines of text.

"You still prefer these old things," she said.

"They don't forget," Prem replied.

She smiled faintly. "Neither do you."

He did not respond.

She left the room with a sense of unease she could not place.

The engagement date was fixed.

A small ceremony first. Families would gather. Nothing extravagant. Madhu's parents wanted simplicity. Arjun agreed. They would plan the rest later.

The announcement traveled.

Congratulations followed.

Prem received one too, from someone who assumed he would be pleased.

He thanked them politely.

That evening, he drove to a part of the city he rarely visited. Roads here were narrower, less disciplined. Construction barriers leaned inward, half-forgotten. Streetlights flickered uncertainly.

He did not linger. He did not stop.

He returned home before midnight.

At the estate, the birds slept. The garden lay still. The pool reflected nothing but darkness.

Prem sat at his desk and removed the half-filled sheet from the typewriter. He placed it carefully in a folder, closed it, and locked the drawer.

He rolled in a fresh page.

This time, he typed without pause.

Not about Arjun.

About sequence.

Outside, Madhu looked at engagement photos on her phone, smiling softly. She imagined her life folding neatly into place, guided by affection and mutual choice.

She felt watched only in the way everyone feels watched by time when the future begins to announce itself.

She did not know that patience had already reached its limit.

And Prem, finishing the page, did not doubt the path ahead.

He had never confused waiting with uncertainty.

Waiting, to him, had always been a form of control.

Chapter Six
The Day That Chose Itself

The day did not announce its importance.

It arrived like any other, sliding into the city with a pale sky and unfinished promises. Traffic thickened early. Horns spoke the same language they always did. People moved with the mild irritation that came from knowing the day would resist them in small ways.

Arjun woke before his alarm.

He lay still for a moment, listening to the fan turn the air without cooling it much, thinking about nothing in particular. There were days when work crowded his thoughts before he even opened his eyes. This was not one of them. The engagement had steadied him. The future had shape now. Even the problems at work felt temporary.

He checked his phone.

A message from Madhu waited.

Did you sleep?

He smiled and typed back.

Like a stone.

She replied almost immediately.

Liar.

He laughed quietly, careful not to wake his roommate. He got ready without hurry, dressed, packed his bag, and stepped out into the morning.

The city met him halfway.

The road outside his building was already busy. A bus lurched forward, stopping abruptly. A vendor shouted prices to no one in particular. Arjun waited for a gap, then merged into traffic, settling into the familiar rhythm of movement and pause.

He liked driving. It gave him time to think without being interrupted. He kept his phone in the compartment, out of reach. Madhu teased him for that, said he was too disciplined. He had shrugged and said some habits were easier to keep than to explain.

At a signal, he stopped and glanced at the time.

He was early.

He sent Madhu a quick message.

Coffee later?

After work.

She responded with a heart.

The signal changed. He moved.

Across the city, Prem woke at his usual hour.

He showered, dressed, and ate breakfast without deviation. His mother joined him at the table, her movements slower these days, more deliberate. She watched him carefully, as she always had, but said nothing.

"Will you be late," she asked.

"Yes," Prem replied.

She nodded. "Don't forget to eat."

"I won't."

He left the house, drove himself, and entered the city as if it were an extension of his office.

Prem did not think about Arjun that morning.

Not consciously.

He thought about timing. About sequence. About how certain days carried weight without asking for it. He had learned long ago that effort was not what decided outcomes. Alignment was.

At the office, his juniors worked quietly. A clerk brought him files. Prem reviewed them efficiently, making brief notations where needed. One case concluded neatly. Another required postponement.

At midday, he stepped out for a short drive.

He did not go anywhere specific.

He moved through parts of the city that did not ask questions. Roads under repair. Signals that lagged. Junctions where lanes dissolved into suggestion. He observed the way people adapted instinctively, the way impatience rewrote rules.

He returned to his office and resumed work.

Nothing in his behavior marked the day as different.

Arjun finished his meetings by late afternoon. Work had gone well. A deployment issue resolved itself sooner than expected. He felt light, unburdened. He packed his bag and left the building, stepping into the humid evening with relief.

Traffic had thickened.

He merged slowly, patient, accustomed to delay. The radio played softly, a voice discussing road conditions somewhere else. He turned it down.

At a junction he passed every day, traffic slowed more than usual. Construction barriers leaned inward, narrowing space. A traffic policeman gestured mechanically, his attention divided between streams of movement.

Arjun eased forward.

He checked the mirror.

Nothing unusual.

A motorbike cut across suddenly, forcing him to brake gently. He allowed it, waited, moved again. He was not in a hurry.

Somewhere behind him, a horn blared. Another answered. The sound spread briefly, then settled.

The city did what it always did.

Arjun reached the center of the junction.

The moment did not feel dramatic.

There was no sense of impending disaster, no cinematic pause. Just a compression of sound and movement, a convergence of ordinary impatience.

He reacted instinctively.

The impact came from the side, sharp and unexpected. Metal met metal. The jolt pushed him forward against the seat belt. The car lurched, then stopped abruptly.

For a fraction of a second, there was silence.

Then noise returned all at once.

Voices. Shouts. The hiss of something leaking. A horn stuck in place.

Arjun sat still, hands gripping the wheel. His ears rang. He tried to breathe evenly. Pain surfaced slowly, dull and spreading, as if his body were negotiating how much to reveal.

Someone knocked on the window.

"Are you okay?"

He nodded, though he was not sure.

The door opened. Hands reached in, guiding him out. The ground felt uneven beneath his feet. He sat down hard on the curb, the world tilting slightly.

His phone slipped from his hand and fell to the road.

A siren sounded somewhere far away.

People gathered, drawn by instinct and boredom in equal measure. Phones appeared. Someone spoke to the traffic policeman. Another person argued about who had moved first.

Arjun's vision blurred briefly.

He reached for his phone, fumbled, then pressed call.

Madhu.

The ringing sounded distant, as if it were happening in another room.

The ambulance arrived faster than he expected.

Lights flashed red against unfinished buildings. Paramedics moved with efficient urgency. They asked questions he answered mechanically. Name. Age. Any pain.

They lifted him onto a stretcher. The world narrowed.

The doors closed.

The siren rose and fell as the ambulance pulled away.

Behind it, traffic resumed, bending around the interruption with practiced indifference.

At the edge of the junction, a man stood watching.

He did not step forward.

He did not take out his phone.

He waited until the ambulance disappeared into the flow of the city, then turned and walked back to his car.

He drove away without haste.

At the hospital, Madhu arrived breathless, her hair loose, her bag forgotten somewhere in the chaos of leaving home. She pushed through the doors, searching faces, guided by fragments of information that refused to form a whole.

A nurse directed her to the emergency ward.

Arjun lay on a bed surrounded by machines. Tubes ran from his arms. His face was pale, marked by small cuts that looked unreal against familiar features.

She reached him and took his hand.

"I'm here," she said, though she was not sure he could hear.

His eyes opened briefly. He looked at her, tried to smile.

"Traffic," he murmured weakly.

She nodded, holding back tears. "Don't talk."

The doctor spoke in careful tones. Head injury. Internal bleeding. They needed to operate.

Madhu nodded, her mind clinging to instructions because feelings threatened to overwhelm her.

Hours passed in fragments.

Paperwork appeared. Questions repeated. A police officer asked about the accident. Madhu answered what she could. She waited. She paced. She sat.

Prem arrived quietly.

He spoke to the nurse first, then approached Madhu.

"I heard," he said simply.

She looked up, startled, then relieved. "They're operating."

"I know," Prem replied. "I spoke to the doctor."

That steadiness anchored her. She did not ask how he knew. It felt natural that he did.

They waited together.

The doctor emerged later, his expression careful.

There were complications.

They had done what they could.

Arjun did not regain consciousness.

The words landed without shape.

Madhu listened as if she were being told about someone else. She nodded. She signed where indicated. She answered questions with automatic politeness.

Prem handled what she could not.

He spoke to officials. He explained procedures. He guided her gently from one place to another when her legs refused to cooperate.

By the time Arjun was declared dead, the night had deepened.

Paperwork followed.

The police concluded what everyone expected. Traffic negligence. Unclear responsibility. An unfortunate accident.

Madhu folded the document carefully and placed it in her bag.

She did not question it.

Why would she?

At the estate, Prem's mother waited.

She had heard the car return late. She had heard Prem move through the house with quiet efficiency. She had heard the typewriter later, its rhythm steady, unbroken.

When Madhu arrived, pale and hollowed, Prem's mother understood immediately.

She held her without words.

Later that night, after Madhu had been settled into a room prepared in advance, Prem's mother went to the study.

Prem sat at the desk, the typewriter before him, a finished page resting neatly beside it.

She looked at him for a long moment.

"You're calm," she said.

"Yes," Prem replied.

She nodded slowly, unease threading through her chest. “Sometimes calm comes later.”

“Sometimes it comes when things are resolved,” Prem said.

She did not respond.

She returned to her room and sat on the edge of the bed, listening to the house settle.

Outside, the city moved on.

Inside, something had shifted permanently.

And Prem, closing the drawer with the finished page inside, did not look back.

The day had chosen itself.

He had only recognized it.

Chapter Seven
What the World Agreed On

Morning arrived without ceremony.

Light filtered through the hospital windows, pale and indifferent, resting on floors that had been cleaned too many times to remember what they once held. Madhu sat in the same plastic chair she had occupied through the night, her bag on the floor at her feet, her phone face down in her lap. She had stopped checking it. Messages had come and gone. None of them changed anything.

A nurse walked past and paused. "You should eat something," she said gently.

Madhu nodded without looking up.

The doctor returned with paperwork, his voice careful, practiced. He explained the sequence again, slower this time, as if repetition might soften the shape of the words. Head injury. Internal bleeding. Complications. No fault that could be isolated. These things happened.

Madhu listened. She did not interrupt. She did not argue.

The police officer arrived next, notebook in hand, expression neutral. He asked the same questions he had asked the night before. Where was he coming from. Where was he going. Had there been any dispute recently. Madhu answered in short sentences.

"No."

"No."

"I don't know."

The officer nodded, satisfied. "Traffic conditions were bad. Construction zone. Witnesses gave conflicting accounts. It looks like an accident."

He wrote the word down.

Accident.

Madhu repeated it silently, testing its weight. It settled easily. It explained everything without asking her to think further.

When Prem entered the room, the officer acknowledged him with a brief nod.

"Sir," the officer said. "We're closing this as a traffic mishap. No criminal angle."

Prem nodded. "That seems appropriate."

The officer closed his notebook. "We'll file the report by evening."

After he left, Madhu turned to Prem.

"They're saying it was an accident," she said, as if confirming something uncertain.

"Yes," Prem replied. "That's what it was."

She did not ask how he knew. His certainty steadied her. It gave the day edges.

Arrangements began immediately.

Arjun's family arrived by afternoon. They had traveled from another part of Karnataka, faces drawn, movements hesitant in a city that did not know them. They clung to official explanations, to procedure, to the comfort of forms and signatures that suggested order.

Madhu watched them from a distance.

She did not know how to approach their grief without drowning in her own.

Prem stood beside her when required. He spoke to Arjun's father calmly, respectfully. He explained the process, the timelines, what would happen next. He answered questions without elaboration. He did not speak about responsibility.

The family accepted his words readily. Authority soothed them.

By evening, Arjun's body was released.

Madhu stood back as rituals took over. Flowers. Prayers. Murmured condolences from strangers who would forget the name by the next day.

She did not cry then.

She felt hollow, as if emotion had stepped aside to make room for function.

Prem noticed.

He guided her gently toward the exit when the noise grew too loud, the air too thick.

"You don't have to stay here," he said quietly. "I can handle this."

She nodded, grateful without knowing why.

They drove away from the hospital in silence.

The city slid past the windows, unchanged. Shops opened. Buses stopped. People crossed roads impatiently. Life did not slow to acknowledge her loss.

At the estate gate, the guard stepped aside without being told.

Inside, Prem's mother waited.

She took one look at Madhu and understood everything that had not been said.

She embraced her without hesitation.

"You're safe here," she said softly.

Madhu did not resist.

That night, Madhu slept in a room that felt prepared for her long before she arrived.

Clean sheets. A glass of water by the bed. Curtains drawn just enough to let the moonlight in without exposure.

Downstairs, Prem sat in his study.

The typewriter rested on the desk, a page rolled in, margins set. He typed slowly, deliberately, documenting the day in his own language. Not facts. Sequence.

The sound traveled through the house, steady and precise.

Prem's mother lay awake, listening.

She recognized the rhythm.

It was not agitation.

It was completion.

In the days that followed, the world agreed on its version of events.

Newspapers printed small columns about traffic accidents. A photograph of a damaged vehicle appeared once, then vanished. The police report concluded without footnotes. No investigation extended beyond the obvious.

People said what people always said.

"Unfortunate."

"Wrong place at the wrong time."

"These things happen."

Madhu repeated these phrases when required. They fit easily into conversation, required no explanation.

At her parents' house, her mother hovered, worried. Her father watched quietly, unsure how to help.

Prem visited once.

He spoke to Madhu's parents respectfully, explaining procedures, offering reassurance. He suggested, gently, that Madhu stay at the estate for a while.

"It will be easier for her," he said. "There's space. Quiet."

Her parents hesitated, then agreed. They trusted him. They trusted reputation.

Madhu returned to the estate that evening without resistance.

It felt like relief.

She did not have to answer questions there. She did not have to explain herself. The servants anticipated her needs without asking. Food appeared when she forgot to eat. Tea arrived when her hands trembled.

She began to move through the garden in the afternoons, walking slowly, following paths that did not require decision.

She noticed the birds.

Some flew freely above the boundary wall, cutting across the sky in careless arcs. Others lived in the aviary, bright and contained, their movements limited but their songs unbroken.

She stopped often to watch them.

"They look happy," she said once, uncertain.

Prem stood beside her. "They are well taken care of."

She nodded. "I like seeing birds fly."

"So do I," he replied. "But flying isn't always kindness."

She thought about that later, sitting by the pool, watching the water reflect the sky without distortion.

Prem's mother watched these exchanges quietly.

She did not intervene.

She still believed the accident.

Why wouldn't she.

She had no reason not to.

Prem was attentive, but not intrusive. Calm, but not distant. He allowed Madhu space without absence.

At night, Madhu lay in her room listening to the typewriter downstairs. The sound steadied her. It meant someone was awake. Someone was holding the world together.

She slept better than she had in days.

Prem's mother noticed this too.

She noticed how quickly Madhu adjusted. How naturally the estate absorbed her. How servants treated her as if she had always belonged.

She noticed Prem's satisfaction, subtle but unmistakable.

Still, she did not suspect him.

She had known her son all her life. She knew his control. His patterns. His intensity.

She did not believe he could cross that line.

She believed his obsession, if it existed, would remain contained.

She believed wrong things about the limits of love.

Weeks passed.

Madhu returned to work briefly, then stopped. Her colleagues understood. Leaves were granted without question. Time stretched.

Prem continued his practice uninterrupted.

He won cases.

He dismantled arguments.

He shaped outcomes.

He returned home each night and typed.

The rhythm never faltered.

One evening, Prem's mother stood outside his study, listening.

The typing slowed, then stopped.

A drawer closed.

She entered quietly.

Prem sat at the desk, his expression composed.

"You're settled," she said.

"Yes," he replied.

She nodded. "Good. Everyone needs closure."

He met her gaze briefly, then looked away.

That night, as she lay awake, Prem's mother thought about the boy in the car years ago, watching Madhu ride past on her father's bike.

She dismissed the memory.

Children watched many things.

It meant nothing.

The world had agreed on its version.

She had no reason to question it.

Not yet.

Outside, birds flew freely above the estate, unseen in the darkness.

Inside, the cages remained closed, clean, and quiet.

The estate slept, holding its order intact.

So did Prem.

Chapter Eight
The Recognition That Comes Late

Grief did not arrive all at once.

For Madhu, it came in fragments, small enough to be mistaken for ordinary fatigue. Some mornings she woke convinced she had dreamed everything. Other mornings she remembered before opening her eyes, the weight settling on her chest as if it had always been there.

The estate accommodated her moods without comment.

Breakfast appeared whether she came downstairs early or late. The servants adjusted silently, plates warming, tea refilled, nothing spoken unless spoken to. No one asked how she was feeling. No one tried to distract her. The absence of pressure felt like kindness.

She walked often now.

The garden paths had become familiar. She knew which turn led to the rose beds, which path curved gently toward the pool, which stretch caught the afternoon sun. She walked slowly, sometimes stopping for no reason, letting thoughts rise and dissolve without direction.

Sometimes she cried without warning.

Sometimes she did not feel anything at all.

Prem watched from a distance.

He did not follow her. He did not join her unless she invited him. He understood timing. Presence mattered only when it was not felt as intrusion.

When he did walk beside her, he spoke about neutral things. The weather. A book he had read years ago. A case that had concluded. He never mentioned Arjun unless she did first.

She appreciated that.

At night, the typing continued.

The sound traveled through the house, steady, measured, anchoring. Madhu began to associate it with safety. As long as the keys struck in that familiar rhythm, the world felt contained.

Prem's mother listened too.

She had always listened.

But now, she listened differently.

It began with something small.

One evening, she noticed that Prem returned home earlier than usual. Not dramatically early, but earlier than his established pattern. He did not appear tired. He did not loosen his tie or remove his jacket immediately.

Instead, he went straight to the study.

The typewriter began soon after.

The rhythm was slower than usual.

Even.

Deliberate.

She frowned slightly.

Prem typed quickly when preparing for court. He typed faster when responding to unexpected developments. Slower typing meant something else.

Resolution.

She dismissed the thought.

Later that night, Madhu joined her in the living room.

They sat together in silence, a cup of tea cooling between them.

"You're very kind," Madhu said suddenly.

Prem's mother looked at her. "Kindness is only useful if it helps."

"It does," Madhu said. "Being here helps."

She hesitated, then added, "Prem has been… very steady."

"Yes," she replied. "That's his nature."

Madhu smiled faintly. "He's always been like this, hasn't he"

The question landed unexpectedly.

Prem's mother paused before answering. "He has always preferred certainty."

Madhu nodded, accepting that easily.

But the word stayed with Prem's mother long after Madhu returned to her room.

Certainty.

The next day, Prem handled a case that involved a fatal accident.

It was unremarkable on the surface. A man had died at a work site. Responsibility was dispersed among contractors, supervisors, and circumstance. Prem argued calmly, focusing on procedure rather than emotion. The court listened.

He did not seek acquittal.

He sought ambiguity.

By the end of the hearing, no one could say exactly who was responsible. The matter was deferred, likely to dissolve into settlements and paperwork.

Prem returned home that evening composed, satisfied.

He typed longer than usual.

His mother passed the study twice before stopping.

She stood outside the door, listening.

The sound was unmistakable now.

Not effort.

Not urgency.

Completion.

She remembered the first time she had heard that sound, years ago, when Prem was still a boy and had decided something without consulting anyone. The decision had not been dramatic. It had simply appeared, already formed.

That memory stirred something uneasy in her chest.

She tried to sleep but could not.

Her thoughts returned to small things she had ignored.

How Prem had known which hospital Arjun was taken to before anyone told him.

How he had spoken to officials with a confidence that suggested familiarity rather than reaction.

How he had never once asked what exactly happened at the accident site.

She had assumed composure.

She had assumed strength.

Now, she wondered if it had been something else.

The next morning, she watched Prem at breakfast.

He read the newspaper without turning pages too quickly. He drank his coffee at the same pace he always did. He asked the cook about the menu for the week and nodded once, satisfied.

"You're very settled," she said.

"Yes," Prem replied. "Things are in order."

Her fingers tightened slightly around her cup.

Later that afternoon, she went for a walk alone.

She rarely did that.

The garden paths were quiet. The air smelled faintly of cut grass. She stopped near the aviary, watching the birds move within their limits. Some perched calmly. Others fluttered briefly, then settled.

She thought of Madhu watching birds in the open sky, smiling without reason.

She thought of Prem's explanation.

Preservation.

Protection.

Limits.

The words took on a different shape now.

That evening, she asked Prem a question she had not planned to ask.

"Did you ever notice Madhu before all this," she said casually, as if the thought had just occurred to her.

Prem did not hesitate.

"Yes," he replied. "Of course."

Her breath caught slightly.

"How," she asked.

"We grew up in the same colony," he said. "I've known her for years."

There was nothing false in the answer.

That was what unsettled her.

He did not soften it. He did not qualify it. He did not pretend the knowledge was incidental.

He simply stated it as fact.

She waited for more.

Nothing came.

That night, she lay awake listening to the typewriter.

The rhythm did not change.

It did not falter.

It did not carry doubt.

It carried finality.

Her realization did not arrive as a shock.

It arrived as alignment.

Pieces she had held separately slid into place without resistance.

The boy in the car, watching from behind glass.

The young man who demanded patterns and control.

The advocate who shaped outcomes without visible effort.

The son who believed rare things needed limits.

And the accident that resolved an obstacle too cleanly, too completely.

She did not think the word murder.

She thought decision.

The next morning, she did not confront him.

She watched Madhu instead.

Madhu moved through the estate with growing ease now. She laughed softly at something a servant said. She lingered near the aviary, speaking to the birds as if they understood.

She looked calmer.

Safer.

That safety frightened Prem's mother more than grief ever could.

That evening, she stood beside Prem in the study.

The typewriter was silent.

"You've done a lot for her," she said.

"Yes," Prem replied.

"She trusts you."

He looked up then, his gaze steady. "She needs stability."

"And you believe you can give it to her."

"I already have."

The certainty in his voice left no room for misunderstanding.

Her realization settled fully.

Not because he confessed.

Because he did not need to.

She left the study without another word.

In her room, she sat on the edge of the bed and stared at her hands.

She thought of all the years she had managed his patterns, softened his edges, believed control would remain contained.

She had been wrong about one thing.

Control did not want to remain contained.

It wanted completion.

Outside, birds flew freely beyond the estate wall, their calls faint, fleeting.

Inside, the cages remained intact.

And Prem's mother, for the first time, understood that the accident had not been an interruption.

It had been a correction.

The recognition came late.

But it came whole.

Chapter Nine
The Silence That Decides

Prem's mother did not speak immediately.

Knowing something and naming it were not the same. She had learned that long ago, raising a child who responded to structure more than affection. Naming changed things. It created edges. It demanded consequence.

So she waited.

Waiting had always been her method.

She watched Prem move through the house with the same measured precision, the same quiet authority. He greeted her as he always did, respectful, composed. He asked if she had slept well. He noticed if she ate less than usual. He adjusted nothing outwardly.

That normalcy unsettled her more than any outburst could have.

In the days that followed her realization, she began to notice details she had once absorbed without thought.

Prem never asked Madhu how the accident had happened.

Not once.

He never asked about the junction. About the sequence. About the other vehicle. He never wondered aloud whether it could have been avoided. He spoke only of what came next. Forms. Procedures. Rest.

Closure.

Grief, she knew, was curious. Even disciplined grief circled the moment of loss, replayed it, searched for meaning or fault. Prem did none of that.

He behaved like someone who had already passed that stage.

One afternoon, she joined Madhu in the garden.

Madhu sat on a bench near the boundary wall, a book resting unopened in her lap. She was watching birds cross the sky, free and careless, their wings cutting through the open space beyond the estate.

"I used to think freedom was the most important thing," Madhu said softly, without looking away. "Now I think maybe safety matters more."

Prem's mother felt something tighten in her chest.

"Why do you think that," she asked gently.

Madhu hesitated. "Because freedom didn't protect Arjun."

The words were simple. Honest. And devastating.

Prem's mother said nothing. She reached out and placed her hand over Madhu's briefly. Madhu squeezed it once, gratefully.

That night, Prem's mother did not sleep.

She lay awake listening to the house, to the way it held sound, to the way it absorbed movement. She listened for the typewriter. It did not begin until late.

When it did, the rhythm was familiar.

Too familiar.

She rose quietly and walked to the study.

Prem sat at the desk, a page nearly complete in the machine. He looked up when she entered, unsurprised.

"You're awake," he said.

"So are you," she replied.

He nodded. "I needed to finish something."

She stepped closer, her eyes drawn to the page. She did not read the words. She did not need to. It was the posture, the calm certainty in his hands, that confirmed everything.

"Prem," she said.

"Yes."

"Do you ever think about limits."

He considered the question briefly. "All the time."

"And do you believe there are limits that should not be crossed."

He met her gaze steadily. "I believe limits exist to protect what matters."

Her breath caught slightly.

"Even if that protection harms others."

He did not answer immediately.

"Harm," he said slowly, "is relative. Loss is inevitable. The question is whose loss we accept."

The answer settled heavily between them.

She did not accuse him.

She did not say Arjun's name.

She did not say the word accident.

She simply said, "You decided this, didn't you."

It was not a question.

Prem did not deny it.

He did not confess either.

"I did what was necessary," he said calmly. "I prevented greater damage."

Her hands trembled, just slightly.

"Damage to whom," she asked.

"To Madhu," he replied. "To what she is."

"You don't own her," she said, the words sharp despite her effort to keep them steady.

"I protect her," Prem said. "Ownership is a crude way of putting it."

She stared at him then, really stared, and saw not cruelty, but conviction.

That frightened her more than cruelty ever could.

"You've crossed a line," she said quietly.

"No," Prem replied. "I reached a conclusion."

She shook her head slowly. "You were a boy once who watched a girl ride past on a bike. I thought time would soften that watching."

"It refined it," Prem said.

The honesty of that admission broke something in her.

She stepped back.

"I can't carry this," she whispered. "I can't live with it."

"You don't have to carry anything," Prem said. "You only have to stay silent."

She looked at him sharply. "Is that what you think this is about. Silence."

"It's about stability," he said. "For everyone."

She laughed softly, a sound without humor. "You sound like your father in court."

He did not react.

"I should tell someone," she said, though even as she spoke, she knew she would not.

"No," Prem said gently. "You shouldn't."

"Why," she asked, her voice breaking now.

"Because it would destroy Madhu," he said. "And it would destroy you. And it would not bring him back."

She sank into the chair opposite the desk, suddenly exhausted.

"You've thought this through," she said.

"Yes."

"Then you've already decided what happens to me."

Prem's expression did not change.

"You are my mother," he said. "I will take care of you."

The words sounded like comfort.

They felt like confinement.

In the days that followed, Prem's mother withdrew.

She stopped walking in the garden. She ate little. She spent long hours in her room, the curtains drawn just enough to let in light without inviting the outside world. She avoided Madhu, not out of anger, but out of fear.

She saw now how easily Madhu had settled into the estate's order.

How safety had replaced freedom without protest.

How grief had softened into dependence.

Prem noticed his mother's withdrawal.

He adjusted the house accordingly.

Medicines appeared on her bedside table without explanation. Meals were lighter, tailored to what she could manage. Servants checked on her more frequently, their concern genuine but guided.

She did not resist.

Resistance would have required energy she no longer had.

One evening, she called Prem to her room.

He came immediately.

"You won't stop," she said.

"No," Prem replied.

"You won't ever let her go."

"No."

She closed her eyes.

"Then you will always be watching," she said. "And she will never know."

"That is how it should be," Prem said. "Knowledge would only hurt her."

Tears slipped from the corners of her eyes, unacknowledged.

"You were my child," she whispered. "I thought love would teach you mercy."

"Love taught me precision," Prem said softly.

She did not answer.

Her health declined quietly after that.

Doctors were called. Explanations offered. Stress. Age. Weakness. No single cause. No urgency. No suspicion.

Prem managed everything.

He drove her to appointments himself. He spoke to doctors with the same composed authority he used in court. He ensured she was comfortable, monitored, protected.

She did not improve.

Madhu noticed, eventually.

"She seems tired," Madhu said one afternoon. "Is she alright."

"She needs rest," Prem replied. "She's carried too much for too long."

Madhu nodded, accepting the explanation.

When Prem's mother died, it was peaceful.

In her sleep, they said.

The house mourned quietly.

Condolences arrived. People spoke of what a good woman she had been. Of how devoted she was to her son. Of how tragic it was that Prem was now truly alone.

Sympathy gathered around him naturally.

Madhu held his hand through the rituals, through the quiet prayers, through the silences that followed.

"I'm here," she said.

Prem believed her.

That night, after the house had settled, Prem returned to the study.

He placed a fresh sheet into the typewriter.

The sound began again, steady and precise.

Outside, birds flew freely in the dark, unseen.

Inside, the estate held its order.

And Prem, alone now in the way that mattered, continued exactly as he had intended.

The silence had decided.

Chapter Ten
Night Belongs to the Estate

The estate changed after sunset.

During the day it appeared disciplined, almost formal, as if it existed to be inspected. Lawns showed their edges. Paths revealed their intention. The boundaries felt reasonable, even generous. Daylight made everything appear explainable.

Night erased explanation.

When darkness settled, the estate withdrew from the world completely. The boundary walls disappeared into shadow. The city sounds thinned, then dissolved. What remained was the controlled hush of land that answered to only one presence.

Prem waited for this hour.

He had always preferred nights, but after Madhu arrived, that preference hardened into need. Darkness made the estate feel complete, sealed, untouched by the randomness he despised. Nothing accidental happened here at night. Everything moved according to design.

After dinner, Prem rose without announcing it.

"Come," he said gently to Madhu.

She hesitated for a fraction of a second, just long enough to notice her own reluctance, then stood. She told herself she was tired of sitting indoors. That the air would help. That a walk would quiet her thoughts.

They stepped outside together.

The garden lights were low, positioned carefully so they illuminated paths without revealing distance. Trees stood tall and unmoving, their canopies forming a ceiling that hid the sky. The air smelled of damp earth and leaves, a scent that felt older than the house itself.

Madhu walked slightly behind Prem at first.

She always did.

Not because he demanded it, but because the space seemed to arrange itself that way. Paths narrowed subtly when she drew level with him, widened again when she slowed. She noticed this only vaguely, as one notices a recurring dream without naming it.

They walked in silence.

Crickets sang softly. Somewhere water moved, not rushing, just existing. The estate did not sleep. It watched itself.

They reached the far lawn where the deer grazed.

Madhu stopped instinctively.

The deer lifted their heads, alert but not alarmed. Their eyes caught the low light briefly, then relaxed. They recognized the space. They recognized Prem.

"They're beautiful," Madhu whispered, as if sound might startle them.

"They're calm," Prem replied. "That matters more."

"They don't run," she said.

"They don't need to," he answered.

The deer moved slowly, deliberately. Their world was large enough to explore, small enough to understand. Fences existed, but they were disguised as landscape. Trees and hedges guided movement without resistance.

Madhu smiled faintly. "They look free."

Prem watched her closely. "They are safe."

She nodded.

The distinction no longer felt like an argument to her.

They continued walking.

Each night, the walks grew longer. The routes varied slightly, but the destination remained consistent. Prem did not rush. He allowed familiarity to do the work. Repetition softened hesitation more effectively than persuasion ever could.

Madhu noticed how the estate responded to night differently now that she was part of it.

Lights turned on as they approached, then dimmed behind them. Servants were absent without being gone. Privacy was not announced. It was assumed.

Prem spoke more during these walks.

Not about the future. Not about grief. He spoke about design. About how space affected people. How certain environments encouraged calm while others provoked anxiety.

"People underestimate surroundings," he said once. "They think emotions come from inside. Most of them don't."

Madhu listened.

She had studied literature. She understood metaphor. She did not yet understand how completely Prem had built his beliefs into stone and glass.

They reached the glass stair house one night without Prem naming it.

The structure rose quietly among the trees, its walls transparent but unreadable in the darkness. At night, the glass reflected forest instead of revealing interior. From outside, it appeared empty. From inside, the world disappeared.

Madhu stopped at its entrance.

"I've never been here," she said.

"I had it built for evenings," Prem replied.

"For walking?"

"For being," he said.

She hesitated again.

The hesitation was familiar now. It no longer felt like resistance. It felt like a pause she had learned to step through.

Inside, the air was warmer. The glass held the night at a distance. Soft lighting traced the stairs, illuminating form without exposure. The trees pressed close, surrounding the structure, hiding it completely.

Madhu felt as though she had stepped out of the world.

"This place feels… hidden," she said.

"That's the point," Prem replied. "Nothing reaches us here."

They stood near the center of the space.

Prem did not touch her immediately.

He waited.

Waiting was his most practiced skill.

Madhu became aware of her breathing. Of how quiet everything was. Of how safe it felt to be unseen.

When Prem finally reached for her hand, she did not pull away.

His touch was steady, deliberate. Not urgent. Not unsure.

She looked at him, searching for something she could not name.

"You don't have to," he said quietly.

The words felt like permission, not invitation.

She nodded, more to herself than to him.

They moved closer, not abruptly, but with the inevitability that had shaped everything else. His hand rested at her waist. Hers remained uncertain for a moment, then settled against his chest.

The glass reflected their silhouettes faintly, dissolving edges, merging forms with shadow.

Madhu felt herself yielding not to force, but to structure. The space held her. The silence supported her. The night erased doubt.

She closed her eyes.

Later, when she would think back on it, she would not remember details. She would remember sensation. Stillness. The feeling of being contained completely, of nothing outside demanding her attention.

When they emerged from the glass house much later, the estate remained unchanged.

The deer grazed quietly. The birds slept in their enclosures. The paths waited patiently.

Madhu walked back beside Prem, no longer behind him.

Her steps matched his.

At the house, she paused.

"I feel calmer here," she said.

"I know," Prem replied.

That night, Madhu slept deeply.

Prem did not.

He sat in his study long after the house had quieted, the typewriter before him, untouched. He did not need to write. Everything had aligned.

The estate had done its work.

Outside, beyond the boundary wall, birds flew freely under the moon, unseen by those inside.

Within the estate, nothing moved without purpose.

And Prem, standing by the window, understood that the night now belonged entirely to him.

Chapter Eleven
Normalization

Morning arrived gently now.

Madhu noticed it first in her body, not her thoughts. She woke without the familiar jolt of loss, without the sharp intake of breath that usually accompanied remembering. The ceiling above her was unfamiliar but no longer strange. Light filtered through the curtains at an angle she had begun to expect.

She lay still for a moment, listening.

The estate breathed around her.

Somewhere far away, water moved through pipes. Leaves shifted softly as if responding to instructions only they understood. There was no urgency in the air. No demand. The silence did not feel empty anymore. It felt arranged.

She rose and dressed without deciding to.

Her feet followed paths they had learned. Down the corridor. Past the staircase. Toward the back veranda where morning waited quietly.

Prem was already awake.

He always was.

He stood near the glass doors, coffee in hand, looking out at the garden. The deer moved slowly across the lawn, their shapes emerging from the morning mist with calm inevitability. They paused, lifted their heads briefly, then returned to grazing.

Madhu joined him without speaking.

For a while, neither of them said anything.

"I used to wake up thinking I had to survive the day," Madhu said finally. "Now I don't think that way."

Prem did not turn to look at her. "Survival is exhausting," he said. "Stability is easier."

She nodded.

They watched the deer.

One stepped closer to the boundary hedge, then turned away instinctively, guided by a limit it did not see but understood. Madhu followed the movement with her eyes.

"They don't try to leave," she said.

"They've learned where they belong," Prem replied.

The word landed softly.

Belong.

Later, at breakfast, the servants moved around Madhu with quiet confidence. They did not ask what she wanted. They already knew. The cook had adjusted the spice level of her food subtly over the past weeks. The tea arrived at exactly the strength she preferred. Her chair was positioned where the light was gentle.

Madhu noticed these things now.

She did not question them.

Routine had replaced vigilance.

After breakfast, Prem left for work as usual. He did not announce his departure. He did not ask her to stay. He simply left, secure in the knowledge that she would.

Madhu walked the garden alone that morning.

The estate looked different in daylight after the night they had spent together. It felt less expansive, more intimate. Corners she had passed without thought now felt deliberate. Each bench seemed placed to invite pause. Each path guided her forward without asking her to choose.

She reached the aviary and stopped.

The birds stirred at her presence, wings fluttering briefly before settling. She watched them move within their space, colorful, alive, unthreatened.

She thought of the birds she used to watch beyond the colony road, cutting across the sky without pattern, without return.

The memory felt distant now.

She placed her hand against the glass of the aviary. The birds did not recoil. They moved closer.

"They don't seem unhappy," she murmured to herself.

She moved on.

The glass stair house appeared different in daylight.

Transparent now, unmistakable in its intention. Surrounded by trees, it still managed to feel private. The glass reflected green and shadow, refusing clarity from any distance.

Madhu stood there for a long moment.

There was no guilt in her. No confusion.

Only a quiet acceptance that something had shifted.

By afternoon, Prem returned.

He did not come to find her immediately. He washed, changed, and went to his study. The typewriter began soon after, the familiar sound traveling through the house.

Madhu paused mid-step when she heard it.

The sound had become a signal. It told her where he was. What state he was in. It told her that the world was being handled.

She sat on the couch and listened.

The rhythm was even.

Not hurried.

Not searching.

Finished.

That evening, Prem suggested a walk without framing it as suggestion.

Madhu followed.

They walked the longer route this time, through the section of the estate that bordered the deer enclosure. Twilight settled around them, softening edges. The deer moved closer to the tree line, their shapes blending into shadow.

"They come here at this hour every day," Prem said. "Routine calms them."

Madhu smiled. "You've noticed everything."

"I notice what matters."

She accepted that without irony.

They walked toward the glass house again, but this time Prem did not lead her inside. They stopped just outside it, standing beneath the trees.

Madhu leaned slightly into him.

The gesture surprised her with its ease.

Prem did not react overtly. He simply adjusted his stance, accommodating her weight.

That was how it worked now.

Accommodation without negotiation.

Days began to take on a predictable shape.

Madhu stopped returning to her parents' house altogether. The idea of leaving the estate felt unnecessarily difficult. Her parents visited occasionally, reassured by how calm she appeared, how settled.

"You look better," her mother said once, relief evident in her voice.

"I am better," Madhu replied, believing it.

Prem greeted them politely, spoke reassuringly, answered questions before they fully formed. He explained Madhu's need for rest, for space, for continuity. Her parents trusted him.

They always had.

At work, Madhu requested extended leave. Her supervisors agreed immediately. Prem had spoken to the right people. The process felt seamless.

She did not return to teaching.

Not yet, she told herself.

She spent her days reading, walking, sitting by the pool. The water reflected her face back at her unchanged. The estate preserved her as it preserved everything else.

At night, the walks continued.

Sometimes they ended in the glass house. Sometimes they did not. The outcome mattered less than the ritual.

Madhu's hesitation faded entirely.

Not because it was argued away.

Because it was no longer necessary.

Prem never pressured. Never asked. He allowed patterns to do what force could not.

One night, Madhu said, almost casually, "I don't feel the urge to go out anymore."

Prem did not smile. "That's natural," he said. "The outside is unpredictable."

"Yes," she agreed. "It feels loud."

He nodded. "Noise exhausts rare things."

She did not recognize the phrase as something she had heard before.

It sounded like truth.

Prem's nights grew longer.

He spent more time in the garden after Madhu slept, walking paths he had designed years ago but had never enjoyed as fully as now. The estate at night responded to him. Lights adjusted subtly as he passed. The trees held still. The boundaries disappeared entirely.

This was the hour he loved most.

Madhu belonged to the night now too.

Her sleep deepened. Her dreams simplified. She stopped dreaming of the road where Arjun had died. The image lost its clarity, then its urgency.

Memory softened.

One morning, she stood by the boundary wall watching birds fly freely beyond it.

She watched for a while, then turned away.

Inside the estate, a deer lifted its head and looked at her.

She smiled back.

Belonging, she realized, did not feel like surrender.

It felt like relief.

Prem watched her from the veranda.

He noted the moment.

He always did.

Nothing important escaped him.

And as the estate settled once more into its rhythm, Prem understood that the hardest part was complete.

Madhu no longer resisted the order.

She lived inside it.

Willingly.

Chapter Twelve
The Shape of a Life

Time inside the estate began to lose its edges.

Days no longer announced themselves with urgency or purpose. They arrived softly, folded into one another, stitched together by routine rather than intention. Madhu noticed it first when she stopped counting weeks. She had once measured her life in semesters, deadlines, lesson plans. Now, she measured it in light and shadow. Morning mist. Afternoon warmth. Night walks.

She did not feel trapped.

That was the unsettling part.

She felt relieved.

The estate carried her days without asking her to decide anything. Breakfast appeared when she woke. Lunch arrived whether she remembered hunger or not. Evenings slowed naturally, bending toward dusk without resistance. The servants moved like extensions of the house, not people with wills of their own. Their presence reassured her. Predictability always did.

Prem noticed her comfort before she did.

He had been watching her long enough to recognize shifts invisible to others. He saw how her shoulders relaxed when she walked the longer garden paths. How her steps slowed near the deer enclosure. How she lingered near the aviary less often now, as if something in her no longer needed the reminder of flight.

One morning, he joined her near the boundary wall.

Birds crossed the sky beyond it, sharp against the pale blue. Madhu watched them without the ache she used to feel. She admired them the way one admires something beautiful but distant, like a painting in a museum one does not need to own.

"They travel far," she said.

"Yes," Prem replied. "And they return to nothing."

She did not argue.

They stood there quietly until the birds disappeared from view. Madhu turned back toward the house without looking over her shoulder.

Prem noted the moment.

It mattered.

Her parents visited less frequently now. Not because they were unwelcome, but because Madhu reassured them so effectively. She spoke calmly on the phone. She sounded rested. She spoke of reading, of walks, of quiet. Grief, they believed, was healing naturally.

"You should come home for a few days," her mother suggested once.

"I don't feel ready," Madhu said. "I'm comfortable here."

Comfort was a powerful word.

Her parents did not press. They trusted her judgment. They trusted Prem even more. He spoke to them occasionally, always respectful, always measured, explaining Madhu's need for continuity.

"She's been through a shock," he said. "Too many changes won't help."

They agreed.

Madhu's world narrowed without resistance.

She stopped checking messages from old friends. Not consciously. Replies grew shorter. Delays lengthened. Eventually, conversations dissolved into polite exchanges that required no continuation.

Her books changed too.

She still read literature, but not the kind that unsettled her. She gravitated toward narratives that ended neatly, stories that resolved conflict without ambiguity. Chaos tired her now.

Prem noticed the titles on her bedside table and approved silently.

At night, the estate became theirs entirely.

After dinner, the walks resumed with ritual precision. Same hour. Same pace. Different paths. Prem understood that variation within structure created the illusion of freedom.

Madhu walked beside him now, not behind.

Sometimes she slipped her hand into his without thinking. Sometimes she leaned into his shoulder briefly as they passed beneath the trees. These gestures were small, unconscious, unexamined.

Prem never commented.

He knew better than to name something that was still settling.

The glass house became part of the routine.

Not every night.

Enough nights.

Madhu no longer hesitated at its entrance. The structure had lost its novelty, replacing it with familiarity. Inside, the world felt distant, muffled by glass and leaves. The darkness outside reflected inward, turning transparency into privacy.

Their intimacy deepened without drama.

There were no declarations, no reassurances. Prem did not ask what she felt. He assumed, and his assumption shaped reality. Madhu accepted this without resistance. Being understood without explanation felt like relief.

Afterward, they often stood together in silence, looking out at the darkened trees.

"This place feels unreal," Madhu said once. "Like it exists only for us."

"That's how it was designed," Prem replied.

She smiled.

The estate adjusted itself subtly around their closeness.

Her room changed again. A drawer cleared for her things. Closet space expanded. Her belongings spread naturally, as if the house had always anticipated them. Nothing felt intrusive. Everything felt accommodating.

One afternoon, Madhu realized she had not thought of Arjun in days.

The realization startled her briefly, then passed.

Grief, she told herself, came in waves. This must be one of the calmer ones.

She did not mention it to anyone.

Prem noticed her lightness.

That evening, he suggested a longer walk.

They moved past the deer enclosure, deeper into the estate where paths curved inward, narrowing perception. The deer lifted their heads briefly as they passed, then returned to grazing. Their movements were unhurried, unafraid.

"They trust this place," Madhu said.

"They've learned it won't harm them," Prem replied.

She nodded.

Trust, she realized, came from consistency, not freedom.

Later that night, Prem sat in his study alone.

The typewriter rested on the desk, polished, waiting. He did not begin immediately. He enjoyed these moments of stillness now, the certainty that everything outside this room aligned with his design.

When he typed, the rhythm was slow and deliberate.

He wrote not of events, but of arrangements. Of spaces. Of routines. Of how lives settled when given the right boundaries.

He stopped midway, satisfied.

Madhu slept deeply upstairs.

Dreams had changed for her. They were quieter now. No sirens. No roads. No sudden loss. She dreamed of gardens, of shaded paths, of animals moving calmly within reach.

She woke without fear.

In the weeks that followed, Prem's presence in her life solidified further.

He began to accompany her to places outside the estate occasionally. Short drives. Controlled environments. Quiet cafés during off hours. Bookstores where no one lingered too close.

Madhu felt a flicker of anxiety each time they left the estate. The city felt loud now. Disordered. People moved unpredictably, spoke too quickly, looked too long.

She clung to Prem's calm during these outings, relieved when they returned.

"I don't know how I used to live here," she said once as they drove back through traffic.

Prem said nothing.

The estate gate closed behind them with its familiar sound, and Madhu felt her shoulders relax.

One evening, Madhu stood near the pool watching the water reflect the fading sky. The surface remained perfectly still.

"I used to think life needed movement," she said. "Now I think stillness is better."

"Movement wastes energy," Prem replied. "Stillness preserves it."

She smiled, satisfied.

Later, she surprised herself by asking, "Do you ever miss the world outside"

Prem looked at her steadily. "No."

She considered her own answer.

"No," she said finally.

The word settled easily.

Her parents called less often now. When they did, Madhu reassured them quickly, efficiently. She sounded content. They had no reason to worry.

She did not return to teaching.

Not because she decided not to.

Because the idea no longer occurred to her with urgency.

Her life had taken a shape that did not require external validation.

One night, as they walked beneath the trees, Madhu stopped suddenly.

"What if I never leave this place," she said, half joking.

Prem turned to face her.

"Why would you need to," he asked calmly.

She searched her own mind for an answer and found none.

They continued walking.

Inside the glass house later, Madhu rested her head against his chest, listening to his steady breathing.

"I feel… held," she said quietly.

Prem's hand rested at her back, firm, reassuring.

"That's because you are," he replied.

Outside, beyond the estate walls, birds flew freely through the night air, guided by instincts that demanded movement.

Inside, Madhu slept without dreaming of flight.

Her life had taken its shape.

And Prem, standing by the glass wall watching the darkness reflect back at him, knew that the transformation was complete.

What remained was simply continuation.

Chapter Thirteen
The World Outside the Gate

The estate had taught Madhu how to be quiet.

Not silence exactly, but a softer way of existing, one that did not collide with other people's urgency. Inside the boundary walls, even sound seemed to know where it belonged. Footsteps softened on stone. Voices lowered instinctively. Doors closed without argument. Nothing demanded to be heard.

Outside the gate, the world had not learned that discipline.

Madhu realized this the first time Prem suggested they attend a public event together.

It was not a celebration, not something loud or intimate. A formal gathering connected to Prem's profession, a dinner attended by colleagues, judges, senior advocates. Safe, controlled, respectable. Prem explained it without persuasion, as if attendance were merely a matter of sequence.

"You should come," he said. "People already expect you to be there."

That sentence stayed with her.

Not want.
Not invite.
Expect.

She agreed before questioning why.

That evening, as she dressed, she felt a faint unease she could not immediately place. The mirror reflected her face clearly, unchanged, yet something about the act of preparing to leave the estate felt unfamiliar. Her hands hesitated over jewelry, over color, over choice.

Prem noticed.

He stepped into the room, adjusted a small detail she had overlooked, smoothed a crease without asking.

"You look fine," he said. "You don't need to think so much."

She smiled, relieved by the instruction.

The drive into the city felt longer than she remembered.

Traffic pressed close. Horns intruded without apology. People crossed roads unpredictably, unconcerned with order. Madhu felt her body tighten slightly, her senses overwhelmed by the lack of containment.

Prem drove calmly, unbothered. His presence grounded her. She watched his hands on the steering wheel, steady, controlled, and let herself relax into that certainty.

At the venue, people recognized him immediately.

Greetings followed. Respectful nods. Subtle deference. Prem moved through the space with practiced ease, introducing Madhu with brief, precise words. No explanations. No embellishments.

"This is Madhu."

That was all.

She noticed how people looked at her.

Not openly. Not rudely.

Evaluating.

Measuring.

She responded as she had learned to inside the estate. Calm. Polite. Reserved. She did not speak more than necessary. She did not offer details.

Prem stayed close.

He guided conversations away from personal topics, redirected questions before they settled. When someone asked about her work, he answered smoothly, framing her absence from teaching as temporary rest.

"She's been through a lot," he said. "We're prioritizing stability."

No one questioned that.

They assumed authority where it was spoken confidently.

Madhu felt something loosen inside her.

The evening passed without incident, but not without impact.

On the drive back, she exhaled deeply.

"I forgot how loud everything is," she said.

Prem glanced at her briefly. "The world isn't designed for people who notice too much."

She nodded. "I don't think I belong there anymore."

The words surprised her with their certainty.

Prem did not respond immediately.

He waited until the estate gate came into view, until the familiar curve of the driveway erased the city from sight.

"Belonging isn't about where you came from," he said then. "It's about where you're safest."

The gate closed behind them.

Madhu felt relief wash through her, immediate and undeniable.

Inside the estate, the air felt different. Softer. Predictable. The lights guided them home without glare. The trees stood exactly where they always had. Nothing had shifted in her absence.

She realized, with a quiet clarity, that the estate had become her reference point.

Everything else now felt temporary.

In the days that followed, Prem began to structure her external life with greater care.

He suggested specific times for outings. Chose places where crowds were minimal. Scheduled visits when the city moved slower. Each decision felt considerate, thoughtful.

Madhu did not resist.

Why would she, when every choice seemed to protect her from discomfort she could no longer tolerate?

One afternoon, her mother called unexpectedly.

"I was thinking of coming by tomorrow," she said. "Just for a few hours."

Madhu hesitated.

The thought of the estate being disrupted unsettled her. Not because she did not love her mother, but because the estate had taught her a different rhythm, one that did not accommodate unpredictability easily.

"Maybe another day," Madhu said gently. "Prem has work, and I'm feeling a bit tired."

Her mother paused. "You've been tired for a long time."

Madhu frowned. "I'm healing."

"I know," her mother said softly. "I just worry."

"There's nothing to worry about," Madhu replied. "I'm happy."

The word sounded convincing even to her.

They ended the call politely.

Madhu sat for a long moment afterward, unsettled by the conversation. Not by what had been said, but by the faint irritation she had felt at the interruption.

She walked into the garden to calm herself.

The deer grazed quietly, lifting their heads briefly as she approached. She watched them move, their behavior unchanged, unaffected by visitors, phone calls, or concern.

They existed entirely within their environment.

Madhu envied that.

Later that evening, Prem joined her.

"You handled that well," he said.

"What," she asked.

"The call," he replied. "You protected your peace."

She nodded, reassured.

That night, during their walk, Prem spoke more openly than usual.

"People confuse care with intrusion," he said. "They think love means access."

Madhu considered this. "Doesn't it"

"No," Prem said. "Love means responsibility. It means knowing when to limit exposure."

She accepted this without argument.

They walked deeper into the estate, past the deer enclosure, toward the glass house. The structure glowed softly among the trees, its transparency concealed by darkness.

Inside, the space felt familiar now. Safe. Expected.

Madhu did not hesitate.

Their intimacy had become part of the estate's rhythm, as natural as the night itself. There was no urgency, no uncertainty. Only continuity.

Afterward, Madhu rested quietly, her thoughts untroubled.

"I don't think I could live anywhere else now," she said softly.

Prem did not smile. "You don't have to."

Days turned into weeks.

Madhu's connections to the outside world thinned further.

Friends stopped calling when replies grew delayed and distant. Her parents adjusted to her unavailability, assuming time would eventually change things. Work faded into memory, something she once did rather than something she might return to.

Her identity simplified.

She was no longer a teacher on leave, a daughter recovering, a woman between lives.

She was simply here.

Prem observed these changes with quiet satisfaction.

Not triumph.

Completion.

One morning, he suggested something new.

"We should formalize things," he said over breakfast.

Madhu looked up. "Formalize"

"Stability helps," Prem replied. "It reassures people. It removes questions."

She considered this.

Marriage had once been a plan with Arjun, something discussed casually, optimistically. The memory felt distant now, softened, lacking urgency.

"With us," Prem added, "nothing would change."

That was what convinced her.

Nothing changing sounded like peace.

She nodded. "Alright."

Prem did not announce it to anyone immediately.

He never rushed outcomes.

He allowed the idea to settle first, to become inevitable before it was spoken aloud.

That afternoon, Madhu stood again by the boundary wall.

Birds crossed the sky beyond it, their wings slicing through open air. She watched them briefly, then turned away.

Inside the estate, the deer moved closer, unafraid.

She stepped toward them instead.

Prem watched from the veranda, noting the direction of her choice.

The world outside the gate continued as it always had, chaotic, loud, unconcerned.

Inside, a life had been shaped carefully, deliberately, into something that no longer questioned itself.

Madhu no longer felt the absence of freedom.

She felt the presence of order.

And Prem, observing the balance he had created, understood that the final transformation did not require force or persuasion.

It required time.

Time, given the right boundaries, always chose correctly.

Chapter Fourteen
Formalities

The word settled into Madhu's life without resistance.

Formalize.

It did not feel heavy. It did not feel final. It felt like a clarification, a smoothing of edges that had already begun to blur. Prem did not present it as a turning point. He mentioned it the way one mentioned a necessary repair, a step that would make everything quieter.

In the days that followed, nothing changed outwardly.

That was the brilliance of it.

Breakfast still arrived at the same hour. The servants moved with the same careful efficiency. The garden paths remained open and inviting. The deer grazed where they always had. The birds sang within their spaces, bright and contained.

Madhu noticed how easily the idea slipped into her routines. She found herself imagining small adjustments without excitement or fear. Where certain things would go. How certain rooms would be used. Who would need to be informed, and who would not.

Prem did not rush her.

He never rushed outcomes.

He allowed the thought to breathe, to settle into her mind until it felt less like a decision and more like recognition.

One afternoon, Madhu sat with Prem's mother's old photo album in the living room. It had been placed there deliberately, she realized later, but at the time it felt like coincidence. The album contained images of a woman whose presence still lingered in the house through absence. Prem's mother smiling at the edge of frames.

Standing beside her son at different ages. Watching him rather than the camera.

Madhu turned the pages slowly.

"She was very composed," Madhu said.

"Yes," Prem replied from the doorway. "She valued order."

"I think she would have liked me," Madhu added, uncertain.

"She did," Prem said without hesitation.

The certainty comforted her.

The estate, too, seemed to accept the idea quietly.

The glass house lights were adjusted slightly, a warmer tone introduced at night. The path leading to it was cleared more carefully, leaves removed before they could accumulate. The space became not just a retreat, but a place with intention.

Madhu did not question these changes.

They felt thoughtful.

Her parents called again.

This time, Prem answered.

He spoke calmly, reassuringly, explaining Madhu's need for stability, her desire to remain in a controlled environment for a while longer. He did not mention marriage. He did not need to. He allowed reassurance to precede revelation.

Madhu listened from the next room, the sound of Prem's voice steady and composed.

Her parents trusted him.

They always had.

When Prem suggested a small visit, brief and contained, Madhu agreed. She felt prepared, insulated by the estate's order.

Her parents arrived one afternoon.

They looked around carefully, noticing the size, the quiet, the way everything seemed maintained without effort. Madhu's mother smiled, relieved by what she saw. Her father nodded approvingly at the calm.

"You seem settled," her mother said.

"I am," Madhu replied.

They spoke of ordinary things. Health. Weather. Distant relatives. Madhu answered easily, her voice steady. She did not feel the need to explain herself.

Prem joined them later, speaking respectfully, listening carefully, offering tea at the right moment. He guided the visit without appearing to.

When her parents left, Madhu felt a familiar sense of relief.

Not because she did not love them.

Because unpredictability tired her now.

That evening, Prem suggested a walk earlier than usual.

The sky was still faintly lit, the transition between day and night slow and deliberate. The estate responded as it always did, lights adjusting, shadows lengthening.

They walked past the deer enclosure.

One of the deer stepped closer to the path, its eyes alert but calm. Madhu paused, instinctively reaching out her hand. The deer did not retreat.

"They trust you," Prem said.

Madhu smiled. "They're gentle."

"They are," Prem agreed. "They thrive here because nothing startles them."

She nodded, understanding without analysis.

They continued toward the glass house.

Inside, the space felt warmer now, less transitional. It no longer felt like a place visited occasionally. It felt like a room that belonged to them.

Madhu rested against the glass wall, watching darkness settle among the trees.

"Do you ever miss chaos," she asked suddenly.

Prem considered the question. "Chaos creates stories," he said. "But stories are exhausting."

She smiled faintly. "I used to love stories."

"You still do," Prem replied. "Just different ones."

Later, when they returned to the house, Madhu noticed something new.

A drawer in the study had been cleared.

Not emptied.

Prepared.

Prem noticed her glance.

"For your things," he said. "When you're ready."

She nodded.

Ready had become a flexible word.

Days passed.

Prem began making small, deliberate introductions. A colleague at a quiet lunch. A family friend at a brief visit. Each interaction was controlled, limited, positive. Madhu was presented as someone cherished, protected, deserving of privacy.

People accepted this narrative readily.

Why wouldn't they.

Madhu noticed how little effort it took now to inhabit this role. She did not have to perform. She did not have to explain. Expectations were minimal. Boundaries were firm.

It felt safe.

One night, Madhu stood alone on the veranda after Prem had gone to his study. The typewriter had not begun yet. The house rested in a rare stillness.

She thought of Arjun then.

Not sharply.

Not painfully.

As a memory softened by distance.

She remembered his voice, his ordinary warmth, his uncomplicated affection. She wondered briefly what life would have looked like had things gone differently.

The question did not trouble her for long.

She did not dwell on it.

The estate had taught her not to linger on possibilities.

Prem joined her a few minutes later.

"You're quiet," he said.

"I was thinking," she replied.

"About what."

"About how things change."

"They do," Prem said. "But change doesn't always mean loss."

She nodded.

He took her hand gently, grounding her.

That night, as they walked through the garden, Madhu felt something she had not felt in a long time.

Certainty.

Not excitement. Not anticipation.

Certainty.

The days that followed moved quickly.

Prem spoke to a lawyer friend quietly. Arrangements were discussed without ceremony. Nothing elaborate was planned. Prem did not like spectacle. He liked legitimacy.

Madhu did not protest.

When Prem told her the date he had in mind, she did not ask why that date. She assumed there was a reason.

"There's no rush," she said.

"There is," Prem replied. "Just not the kind you think."

She accepted that.

Her wardrobe shifted subtly again. Practical items replaced sentimental ones. Her bookshelves changed, titles rearranged, some removed entirely. She did not miss them.

She did not notice when the estate became her address in official records.

Not immediately.

It felt natural when she did.

One evening, Prem returned home earlier than usual.

He did not go to the study. He did not type.

He joined Madhu in the living room and sat beside her.

"I've spoken to your parents," he said.

She looked at him calmly. "About us"

"Yes."

She waited.

"They want to meet," he continued. "To make things proper."

Madhu nodded. "That's reasonable."

Prem watched her closely.

No hesitation.

No fear.

Only acceptance.

That night, Madhu slept deeply.

Dreams came softly, without urgency. She dreamed of the garden at night, the paths lit just enough, the deer moving quietly, the glass house glowing among the trees.

She did not dream of the city.

She did not dream of roads.

Morning arrived as it always did.

And as Madhu stepped out onto the veranda, watching the estate wake into its familiar calm, she realized that the idea of a life beyond the gate now felt abstract.

Possible, perhaps.

But unnecessary.

Prem watched her from the doorway, noting her posture, her ease, her quiet certainty.

Formalities, he knew, were not about change.

They were about recognition.

And recognition, once granted, rarely asked to be undone.

Chapter Fifteen
Consent Without Questions

The meeting with her parents happened on a Sunday afternoon.

Prem chose the time deliberately. Late enough that the city would be subdued, early enough that fatigue would soften insistence. He arranged the seating so no one faced a window directly. He set the tea before anyone asked. The house accepted the visit the way it accepted everything else, by making room without shifting its center.

Madhu sat between her parents, close enough to feel familiar, far enough to feel separate. She noticed the arrangement and did not question it. Her father spoke first, cautiously, respectful of Prem's presence and the quiet authority he carried even while sitting still.

"We've been thinking," he said. "About what's best for her."

Prem nodded once. "So have I."

The conversation unfolded exactly as Prem had anticipated. Concern framed as care. Questions softened into reassurance. Madhu answered when asked, her voice steady, calm, unburdened by the need to persuade.

"I'm settled here," she said simply. "I feel… stable."

Her mother watched her closely, searching for cracks. She found none.

Prem spoke last. He always did.

"We're not rushing anything," he said. "We're formalizing what already exists. Continuity matters."

Her parents exchanged a glance. Continuity sounded reasonable. Stability sounded kind. The estate itself seemed to support the argument, quiet and composed, a visible promise of protection.

They agreed.

Not enthusiastically. Not reluctantly.

They agreed because there was nothing to argue against.

After they left, Madhu felt lighter.

She walked with Prem through the garden, her steps easy, her thoughts untroubled.

"I thought I would feel nervous," she said. "I didn't."

"That's because there was no conflict," Prem replied. "Conflict comes from competing truths."

She smiled faintly. "There aren't many truths anymore."

He did not correct her.

The days that followed moved with renewed certainty.

Formalities progressed quietly. Documents were prepared. Appointments scheduled. Everything happened through channels that did not demand Madhu's presence. Prem believed in removing friction wherever possible. She would be informed when something required her acknowledgment. Nothing required her input.

This did not trouble her.

She trusted his judgment.

She trusted his sense of order.

One afternoon, Madhu noticed that her teaching certificates had been moved from her drawer to a file in the study. Not hidden. Archived. She stood for a moment, considering whether to retrieve them.

She did not.

The glass house became their place of evenings now.

Not occasionally.

Routinely.

After dinner, they walked. Sometimes past the deer enclosure, sometimes beneath the taller trees where light barely reached the ground. The paths felt narrower now, more intimate, as if the estate itself were guiding them inward.

Inside the glass house, Madhu felt a calm that bordered on detachment. The outside world reflected back at her as shadow and silhouette. Nothing intruded. Nothing demanded.

Prem's presence felt inevitable there.

She no longer hesitated.

Consent had become less about decision and more about alignment.

They did not speak much during these moments. Words felt unnecessary. The space held meaning without explanation.

Later, as they stood together watching darkness pool beneath the trees, Madhu said something that surprised even her.

"I don't remember the last time I made a choice."

Prem turned slightly, attentive but not alarmed.

"Choice is overrated," he said. "Most people are burdened by it."

She nodded, relieved by the permission implicit in his words.

The estate responded to her acceptance.

Her routines deepened. Meals arrived at the same time daily. Walks followed familiar arcs. Nights ended in predictable silence. The typewriter's sound returned as a constant, a low hum of certainty that accompanied her sleep.

She began to associate that sound with safety.

One night, she woke briefly, disoriented. The room was dark, the house quiet.

Then she heard it.

The keys striking metal. Steady. Measured.

She relaxed instantly and returned to sleep.

In the weeks leading up to the formal announcement, Madhu's contact with the outside world diminished further.

Friends stopped calling entirely. Messages went unanswered long enough to dissolve on their own. Social media became irrelevant. She deleted apps without ceremony, not as an act of withdrawal, but as one might remove clutter.

Her parents visited once more.

This time, Madhu guided the visit herself. She offered tea, suggested a walk, spoke confidently about her plans. Her mother watched her closely, unsettled by the ease with which she occupied this life.

"You've changed," her mother said gently.

Madhu smiled. "I've simplified."

Her father nodded, satisfied.

Prem joined them briefly, then excused himself. He allowed Madhu to host. He had already secured what mattered.

After they left, Madhu felt no lingering emotion.

She did not feel loss.

She felt closure.

That night, as they walked beneath the trees, Prem spoke more directly than he had in weeks.

"People will expect certain things," he said. "After the announcement."

Madhu considered this. "Like what."

"Appearances. Participation. Questions."

She frowned slightly. "I don't like questions."

"I know," Prem replied. "That's why I'll handle them."

She exhaled, relieved.

"I want things to stay like this," she said. "Quiet."

"They will," Prem said. "As long as we don't invite noise."

She nodded, trusting him completely.

The announcement was made without spectacle.

A few calls. A few messages. A small gathering planned for legitimacy rather than celebration. Prem did not like crowds. He preferred acknowledgment without attention.

Madhu's name appeared alongside his in formal contexts now. Documents. Invitations. Records.

She noticed this vaguely, as one notices a change in weather without marking the day.

The estate adapted again.

Her room shifted subtly, merging into Prem's space without declaration. Drawers were shared. Closets combined. Her belongings lost their separation naturally.

She did not resist.

Resistance would have required desire.

Desire had been replaced by ease.

One evening, Madhu stood near the aviary, watching the birds move within their space. Their feathers caught the low light, vibrant and alive.

She felt no urge to open the enclosure.

"They seem content," she said.

"They are," Prem replied. "They don't need to choose anymore."

She smiled, comforted.

At the deer enclosure, the animals moved closer as she approached. One lifted its head, alert but calm. Madhu reached out, her fingers brushing its neck briefly. It did not flinch.

"They trust this place," she said.

"They trust consistency," Prem corrected.

She accepted that.

As the days passed, Madhu's identity continued to refine itself.

She stopped referring to herself as a teacher. She did not correct people when they spoke of her as Prem's partner, soon to be wife. The distinction no longer mattered to her.

She felt held within a narrative that did not require her to explain herself.

One afternoon, she found an old notebook in a box of her things. Notes from her M.A. course. Margins filled with questions, arguments, reflections.

She flipped through it briefly.

The questions felt distant. The arguments unnecessary.

She placed the notebook back in the box and closed it.

That night, Prem did not go to the study.

He joined Madhu in the garden instead.

They walked without destination, their steps slow, synchronized. The estate at night felt smaller now, more intimate, as if the boundaries had drawn closer to them.

"You're quiet," Prem said.

"I feel complete," Madhu replied.

He stopped walking and turned to face her.

"Completion is rare," he said. "It should be protected."

She nodded.

Inside the glass house later, Madhu rested her head against his shoulder.

"I don't feel like I'm choosing you," she said softly. "I feel like I'm where I'm supposed to be."

Prem's hand rested firmly at her back.

"That's what choice looks like when it's done correctly," he said.

Outside, the trees pressed close, shielding the glass from any distant light. The estate held its breath, its order intact.

Beyond the walls, the world continued its unpredictable movement. Roads filled. Lights flickered. People hurried toward destinations that shifted as soon as they arrived.

Inside, Madhu felt none of that pull.

Her life had narrowed into something manageable, something quiet.

Consent had become unnecessary.

Everything important had already been decided.

And Prem, standing with her in the center of the space he had designed for this exact moment, understood that there would be no reversal.

There was no longer a door to walk back through.

There was only continuation.

And continuation, once accepted, required no questions at all.

Chapter Sixteen
After the Gate Closes

The announcement passed through the world with very little resistance.

That was what surprised Madhu most.

She had expected questions, objections, at least curiosity sharp enough to sting. Instead, people accepted the news with a calm that mirrored her own. Messages arrived framed in approval. Voices on the phone softened into reassurance. Even those who had once known her differently adjusted quickly, as if her new place in the world clarified something that had always been ambiguous.

Prem understood this better than she did.

People, he knew, preferred finished stories.

An unmarried woman in grief invited concern, speculation, advice. A woman settled into a respected man's life required none of that. Formality removed uncertainty. It gave others permission to step back.

Madhu felt the effect immediately.

Calls from acquaintances stopped entirely. Her parents spoke with relief now, their questions replaced by practical details and future planning. Her mother asked about dates, clothing, rituals. Her father asked about legalities and arrangements. Madhu answered when asked, briefly, efficiently, then handed the phone to Prem when things became complex.

He handled everything.

The estate absorbed this new phase without effort.

Spaces adjusted again, not dramatically, but decisively. Madhu's room ceased to be hers alone. Her clothes moved fully into Prem's space.

Drawers that had once been temporary became permanent without ceremony. The house no longer treated her as a guest.

It treated her as fixed.

Madhu noticed this one morning when she went looking for something and found it already where it should have been, placed there without her asking. She stood for a moment, holding the object, surprised not by the action but by how natural it felt.

Someone had thought ahead for her.

That thought comforted her.

The days took on a quieter confidence now.

Madhu no longer wandered the garden aimlessly. Her walks had purpose, even if she could not have named it. She favored certain paths, avoided others, moved through the estate with the familiarity of someone who belonged to it rather than visited.

The deer recognized her instantly now.

They no longer lifted their heads in alert curiosity when she approached. They continued grazing, secure in her presence. One of them followed her briefly one afternoon, stopping a few steps behind her before losing interest.

Madhu smiled at the small gesture.

"They know you," Prem said, watching from a distance.

"They're not afraid," she replied.

"They don't need to be," he said.

The statement settled between them easily.

At night, the estate became even quieter than before.

Prem's love for the darkness had always existed, but now it sharpened. Night no longer represented solitude. It represented completeness. The absence of interruption allowed him to experience the estate as it was meant to be experienced.

Private.

After dinner, the walks continued, but the tone shifted subtly.

They no longer felt exploratory.

They felt owned.

Madhu noticed that Prem rarely asked where she wanted to walk anymore. He chose the path and she followed without resistance, trusting that he knew where they were going even when she did not.

Trust, she had learned, reduced effort.

The glass house remained their center.

Inside it, time felt suspended. The outside world reflected back only darkness and trees, the glass dissolving boundaries until it felt like the structure existed nowhere at all. Madhu no longer felt self-conscious there. She did not think of how it looked from outside, or whether anyone could see them.

No one could.

The estate had been designed to ensure that.

One night, as they stood together in silence, Madhu spoke without turning to him.

"I don't feel watched anymore," she said.

Prem's gaze sharpened slightly. "Did you before."

"Yes," she replied. "All the time. By expectations. By people. By myself."

"And now."

"Now I feel invisible," she said, and then corrected herself. "No. Seen. But only by you."

Prem did not respond immediately.

That was exactly the balance he had engineered.

In the days that followed, Prem began withdrawing Madhu from the last remnants of her old life.

Not abruptly.

Not visibly.

He did it the way he did everything else.

Through replacement.

Her teaching materials were archived fully now, moved into labeled boxes and stored in a room she rarely entered. Her books were reorganized. Some disappeared quietly, replaced by others he knew she would find calming, narratives without unresolved conflict.

Her phone changed too.

Not the device itself, but how it functioned in her life. Notifications dwindled. Contacts thinned. Eventually, it became a tool for logistics rather than connection.

Madhu noticed the silence and welcomed it.

The fewer voices reached her, the lighter she felt.

One afternoon, Prem suggested a drive.

She hesitated instinctively.

The city still unsettled her.

"We won't stay long," he said. "Just enough to remind you that the estate exists because the world does not."

She agreed.

They drove during an hour when traffic thinned, moving through roads that Prem knew would not provoke unpredictability. Still, Madhu felt tension build in her chest as the estate disappeared behind them.

The city pressed in immediately.

Noise. Movement. Disorder.

People crossed streets without looking. Vehicles cut lanes abruptly. Shops spilled sound and color into space that felt too exposed.

Madhu clutched her bag unconsciously.

Prem noticed.

He placed a hand briefly over hers.

"We'll go back soon," he said.

She nodded, grateful.

At a quiet café, they sat for a short while. Prem chose the table, the timing, the exit. Madhu drank her tea quickly, her eyes drawn constantly to the door.

When they returned to the car, she exhaled in relief.

"I don't belong out here anymore," she said as they drove back.

Prem did not correct her.

The estate gate closing behind them felt like a physical release.

Madhu leaned back in her seat, exhausted.

"I don't know how I lived like that," she murmured.

"You adapted," Prem said. "Now you don't have to."

That night, Madhu slept deeply, the kind of sleep that erases dreams.

Prem remained awake.

He walked the estate alone after Madhu had gone to bed, moving through spaces he had designed and refined over years. The deer slept near the tree line, barely visible. The birds remained quiet within their enclosures. The glass house reflected only darkness.

Everything was where it should be.

He paused near the boundary wall and looked outward, toward the city lights barely visible beyond trees and distance. He felt no curiosity. No pull. The world outside no longer mattered.

Inside the estate, everything that mattered was contained.

The following weeks passed without disruption.

Arrangements progressed smoothly. Rituals were planned with minimal spectacle. Prem rejected unnecessary tradition. He preferred efficiency to symbolism, control to celebration.

Madhu agreed with everything.

She no longer felt the need to contribute opinions. Agreement came easily now, unburdened by the need to define herself separately.

One evening, she surprised Prem by saying, "I don't think I could survive without this place."

Prem turned to look at her.

"You wouldn't need to," he said. "This place is permanent."

She smiled, reassured.

Later that night, Madhu stood alone by the aviary.

The birds moved softly within their space, their colors muted in the low light. She watched them for a long time, noticing how little they struggled, how familiar their movements had become.

"They don't try to escape," she whispered.

"They don't need to," Prem said, having approached silently behind her. "They have everything they need."

She nodded.

In that moment, she did not feel like one of them.

She felt chosen.

That distinction mattered to her.

The estate continued its quiet work.

Days folded into one another without friction. Madhu's identity narrowed further, refined into something simpler and easier to maintain. She no longer thought of herself in terms of past roles or future possibilities.

She thought only in terms of now.

And now was sufficient.

Prem watched her transformation without emotion.

This was not triumph.

It was confirmation.

He had not forced the outcome. He had only removed noise until truth remained.

And the truth was simple.

Madhu no longer wanted a world that asked her to choose.

She wanted a world that had already decided.

The gate remained closed.

No one asked what lay beyond it.

No one needed to.

Chapter Seventeen
The Last Adjustments

The closer the formal date came, the quieter the estate became.

It was not a silence born of anticipation or anxiety. It was a tightening, a drawing inward, as if the place itself were preparing to seal something permanently. The servants moved with increased precision. Conversations shortened. Even footsteps seemed to learn restraint.

Madhu noticed this without naming it.

She had learned not to name things that felt stable.

Her days followed a predictable arc now. Morning light through the veranda. Breakfast placed without inquiry. A walk through the garden, always beginning the same way, diverging only slightly depending on Prem's presence. Afternoons spent reading or sitting near the pool, the water reflecting a sky she no longer felt compelled to interpret.

In the evenings, Prem returned earlier more often.

Not because his work had reduced, but because it no longer required expansion. His professional life had reached a stage where momentum carried itself. His reputation preceded him. His instructions were followed without explanation. Control, once established, did not need constant reinforcement.

He preferred to be home.

Madhu felt this preference like a quiet compliment.

One afternoon, she wandered into a wing of the house she rarely visited now. It had once held rooms she considered transitional, spaces she passed through without attachment. Now, she found them subtly repurposed. Furniture rearranged. Lighting adjusted. Shelves cleared.

Preparation without announcement.

She stood in one room longer than the others.

It was empty except for a chair placed precisely near the window.

She frowned slightly, unsettled.

When Prem found her there later, he did not ask what she was doing.

"This room will be useful," he said calmly.

"For what," she asked.

"For quiet," he replied. "Sometimes separation improves closeness."

She nodded.

That explanation felt complete.

The estate at night grew more intimate as the days progressed.

Their walks shortened, not because they tired, but because the routes had already done their work. They no longer needed repetition. Familiarity had replaced exploration.

The glass house remained essential.

Madhu noticed how the trees around it had been trimmed recently, not to reveal the structure, but to conceal it further. Sightlines adjusted. Shadows deepened.

"You've changed it," she said one night.

"Yes," Prem replied. "Privacy is most important when things are finalized."

She accepted this without discomfort.

Inside the glass house, their closeness had lost any trace of hesitation. It had become routine, not in the sense of boredom, but in the sense of inevitability. Madhu no longer examined her own responses. She trusted them.

Trust simplified everything.

One evening, Madhu surprised herself by asking a question she had not asked in months.

"Do you ever think about what comes after," she said quietly.

Prem considered the question carefully.

"After what," he asked.

"After… everything is done," she said. "The ceremonies. The expectations."

"There is no after," Prem replied. "There is only maintenance."

She smiled faintly. "That sounds exhausting."

"Only if the structure is weak," he said. "This one isn't."

She leaned into him, reassured.

The mention of ceremonies did not disturb her.

She had stopped associating them with transformation. They felt administrative, not emotional. A recognition rather than a beginning.

Her parents visited once more before the date.

This visit felt different.

Shorter. More formal.

Madhu noticed how her mother's eyes moved through the house, lingering on details, returning to Madhu's face repeatedly. There was concern there, but it was muted by relief.

"You seem… settled," her mother said again.

Madhu nodded. "I am."

Her father spoke mostly to Prem, asking practical questions. Timelines. Legalities. Arrangements. Prem answered with clarity, removing uncertainty before it could form.

The visit ended sooner than expected.

Madhu felt no sadness at their departure.

Only quiet.

That evening, she walked alone in the garden for the first time in days.

The deer lifted their heads briefly as she passed, then returned to grazing. One stood still for a moment, watching her with calm, unreadable eyes.

Madhu stopped.

She studied the animal carefully.

"You don't miss anything, do you," she murmured.

The deer did not respond.

It did not need to.

Later, Prem joined her near the boundary wall.

"You walked alone today," he observed.

"I wanted to," she replied. "Just to see if it felt different."

"And did it."

"No," she said. "It felt the same."

He nodded, satisfied.

The night before the formalities, Prem did not use the typewriter.

This absence of sound unsettled Madhu briefly. She lay awake, listening for the familiar rhythm, then realized what had changed.

Nothing remained to be written.

She rose quietly and walked downstairs.

Prem stood in the living room, lights low, the house stilled around him.

"You're awake," he said.

"So are you," she replied.

He looked at her steadily. "Tomorrow will be busy."

"I know," she said. "I don't feel nervous."

"That's because there's nothing to anticipate," Prem said. "Everything is already in place."

She considered this.

"Do you ever worry," she asked, "that I might change my mind."

The question hung between them, not accusatory, not afraid. Curious.

Prem answered without hesitation.

“No.”

The certainty in his voice did not frighten her.

It calmed her.

“Why,” she asked softly.

“Because people don’t abandon safety,” he replied. “They abandon chaos.”

She nodded.

That night, she slept deeply.

Dreams did not come.

Morning arrived as it always did.

The estate moved into motion smoothly, efficiently. Servants appeared and disappeared. Arrangements unfolded. Nothing felt rushed. Nothing felt ceremonial.

Madhu dressed in silence.

Her reflection showed a woman calm, composed, untroubled. She did not feel like someone about to cross a threshold. She felt like someone acknowledging a fact.

Prem joined her briefly, adjusted a detail, then stepped back.

“You’re ready,” he said.

She believed him.

The formalities themselves passed without incident.

They were smaller than expected. Quieter. Contained within rooms that did not invite spectacle. Words were spoken. Signatures placed. Witnesses nodded.

Madhu followed instructions easily.

Her hand did not tremble.

When it was done, nothing shifted.

That was what struck her most.

The world did not rearrange itself.

The estate did not change.

Prem did not change.

She did not change.

Everything simply continued.

Later that evening, when the last visitor had left and the house settled back into its familiar stillness, Madhu walked through the garden alone.

The air felt exactly the same as it had the night before.

She stood near the glass house, watching the reflection of trees ripple faintly across its surface.

Prem joined her moments later.

"It's done," she said.

"Yes," he replied. "Now it's protected."

She smiled.

"Protected feels right," she said.

They walked together through the estate one last time that night, not marking the occasion, not naming the moment. The paths accepted their footsteps. The trees held their shadows. The deer grazed without fear.

Beyond the boundary wall, the world continued its restless movement.

Inside, nothing asked to be changed.

Madhu realized, with a quiet finality, that she no longer thought in terms of doors or exits.

There was nowhere she wanted to go.

There was only this place, this order, this certainty.

And certainty, once established, did not need to be questioned.

The last adjustments had been made.

Nothing remained undone.

Chapter Eighteen
Life without Edges

Nothing followed the formalities the way Madhu had once imagined life-changing moments would.

There was no surge of emotion, no collapse into relief or fear. The day after looked exactly like the day before. Morning arrived quietly. The estate breathed as it always had. The servants moved with the same practiced silence. The garden held its shape. The deer grazed. The birds sang within their limits.

That sameness calmed her.

Madhu woke later than usual and lay in bed for a while, listening. The house was awake, but it did not intrude. She felt no urgency to rise. No expectation pressed against her chest.

She had not realized how much of her life had once been defined by expectation.

She dressed slowly and walked out onto the veranda. The air was cool, steady. The sky had no intention of surprising her. She noticed how natural it felt now to move through the house without thinking about direction. Her feet chose paths for her. Her hands reached for doors already open.

Prem joined her a little later.

"You slept well," he said.

"Yes," she replied. "I didn't dream."

"That will happen more often," he said. "Dreams come from unrest."

She accepted this without question.

They ate breakfast together in silence. Not the silence of distance, but of completion. The servants cleared plates and refilled cups without being asked. Madhu noticed how seamlessly they addressed her now, how their glances carried acknowledgment rather than inquiry.

She belonged here fully.

The day unfolded without structure, and yet without chaos.

Madhu walked the garden alone, then returned to sit by the pool. The water lay still, reflecting the sky in perfect symmetry. She traced the edge of the pool with her fingers, noticing how even the smallest disturbance rippled outward before settling again.

She liked how quickly things settled here.

In the afternoon, Prem left for a short while.

He did not explain where he was going. He did not need to. Madhu no longer felt the need to track his movements. The idea of waiting had lost its tension. Waiting was no longer a gap to be filled. It was simply a state.

She spent the time organizing a drawer she had never fully unpacked.

Inside were remnants of a life that felt distant now. Old notebooks. Letters. Photographs. She moved through them carefully, not with nostalgia, but with curiosity, as one might examine artifacts from a place no longer inhabited.

She paused at a photograph of herself taken years ago.

She looked younger, but not in the way people usually meant. Her eyes in the picture seemed restless, searching. She remembered the girl she had been then. Ambitious. Thoughtful. Constantly negotiating with the world.

She placed the photograph back into the drawer and closed it.

There was no impulse to keep it out.

When Prem returned, evening had begun to gather. The light softened. Shadows stretched. The estate responded instinctively, lights adjusting, pathways revealing themselves gently.

They walked together after dinner, as they always did.

Madhu noticed something had changed.

Not in Prem.

In herself.

She no longer thought of the walk as something they did. It felt like something the estate required of them, a rhythm that included them without asking permission.

They passed the deer enclosure.

The animals lifted their heads briefly, then resumed grazing. One stood close to the fence, its body angled toward the path. Madhu stopped and watched it for a moment.

"It doesn't even look curious anymore," she said.

"It knows the limits," Prem replied. "Curiosity fades when uncertainty does."

She nodded.

They continued walking.

That night, the glass house felt different.

Not warmer. Not darker.

Smaller.

Not in size, but in necessity.

Madhu stood inside it and realized she no longer needed it to feel safe. Safety had expanded beyond the structure. It existed everywhere within the estate now.

"This place doesn't feel as important as it used to," she said quietly.

Prem studied her carefully. "Why do you think that is."

"Because I don't feel exposed anywhere anymore," she said.

He considered this, then nodded.

"That's how it should be."

The realization settled deeply within her.

The glass house had been a transition.

The estate itself was now complete.

Days passed.

Madhu stopped marking them.

She woke when she woke. Ate when food appeared. Walked when the air felt right. She read occasionally, but less than before. Books felt unnecessary now. Stories created friction. Her life no longer required interpretation.

Prem's work continued without interruption.

He left and returned at predictable hours. His presence remained steady, unremarkable, reassuring. He no longer typed late into the night. The typewriter rested unused, polished and ready but silent.

One evening, Madhu noticed its absence.

"You haven't been writing," she said.

"There's nothing left to organize," Prem replied. "Everything is where it should be."

She felt a wave of calm at his words.

Later that night, she woke briefly and realized something else.

She did not miss the sound.

The house itself had replaced it.

The quiet was complete.

Madhu's parents called less frequently now.

When they did, conversations were brief and pleasant. Madhu answered questions easily, offering reassurance without detail. Her mother's voice carried relief rather than concern. Her father spoke of practical matters only.

They had accepted the shape of her life.

Friends existed now only as names she recognized faintly. She did not think about why she no longer spoke to them. The absence felt natural, like a habit that had simply faded.

One afternoon, Madhu stood near the boundary wall again.

She did this less often now, but the habit had not disappeared entirely. Beyond the wall, birds flew freely, cutting through open space with effortless movement. She watched them for a long moment.

There was no longing in her chest.

Only observation.

She turned away before Prem joined her.

"I used to think freedom looked like that," she said, gesturing vaguely toward the sky.

"And now," Prem asked.

"Now I think freedom is not having to choose where to fly," she replied.

He smiled faintly.

That night, Prem walked the estate alone after Madhu had gone to bed.

He moved slowly, deliberately, as if taking inventory of a life that had finally aligned with his design. The deer slept near the trees. The birds rested within their enclosures. The glass house reflected nothing but darkness and leaves.

Everything was contained.

He paused near the boundary wall, not to look beyond it, but to confirm its presence. The wall did not feel like a barrier. It felt like a definition.

Inside this line, the world made sense.

Inside this line, nothing unexpected could intrude.

He returned to the house and stood for a moment outside the bedroom door, listening to Madhu's steady breathing. He did not enter immediately. He did not need to.

The sound reassured him.

Days turned into weeks.

Madhu's life continued without edges.

There were no decisions that required effort. No choices that produced anxiety. Her identity had simplified into something manageable, something that did not demand articulation.

She was not a teacher who had stopped working.

She was not a woman who had lost a lover.

She was not someone who had chosen one life over another.

She was simply here.

The estate absorbed her completely.

One morning, Madhu realized she could no longer remember the exact moment when her life had crossed from one state into another. The transition had been too gradual, too gentle to mark.

She did not mind.

Sharp lines belonged to a world that hurt.

Here, everything blurred into calm.

She walked the garden one last time that day, alone, moving through paths she could now navigate with her eyes closed. She paused near the deer enclosure and watched them graze.

"They don't wonder," she murmured.

Prem's voice came from behind her. "Wondering is a form of unrest."

She nodded.

They walked back toward the house together, their steps aligned, unhurried.

The estate settled around them, complete and quiet.

Beyond the walls, life continued to rush and fracture and demand.

Inside, Madhu lived without edges.

And Prem, watching her move through the space he had shaped for her, knew that the final state had been reached.

There was nothing left to add.

Nothing left to remove.

Only maintenance.

Only time.

Chapter Nineteen
Maintenance

Maintenance did not announce itself.

It entered quietly, disguised as comfort, as familiarity refined to its smoothest edge. Nothing broke. Nothing resisted. The systems Prem had put in place did not require correction so much as gentle reinforcement, the way one reinforces a path simply by walking it daily.

Madhu woke each morning without anticipation.

That, she realized, was the truest measure of how thoroughly her life had settled. Anticipation implied desire. Desire implied lack. Here, nothing felt lacking.

She moved through the house like a resident who had never lived anywhere else. Doors opened before she reached them. Curtains parted at the right hour. Water warmed at predictable intervals. Even the weather seemed to cooperate, aligning itself into mildness more often than not.

She had stopped asking herself whether this was happiness.

The question felt irrelevant.

Happiness was a word that belonged to comparison. This life no longer compared itself to anything else.

Prem observed her routines with quiet attention.

Not surveillance.

Confirmation.

He noticed the way she paused less often near the boundary wall. The way her gaze lingered longer on the deer than on the sky. The way she no longer startled at unfamiliar sounds because there were no unfamiliar sounds left.

The estate had trained her senses.

That evening, as they walked the garden, Madhu said something unexpected.

"I don't think I could live in a smaller place."

Prem looked at her carefully. "Why."

"It would feel… exposed," she said. "Like walls too close together would trap thoughts."

He nodded. "Space prevents reflection."

She accepted that explanation easily.

They passed the deer enclosure, their steps slowing instinctively. The animals moved closer to the tree line as dusk settled, their shapes blurring into shadow. One lifted its head and watched them pass, calm, uninterested.

Madhu felt a strange kinship in that indifference.

Later that night, Prem returned briefly to the study.

Not to write.

To check.

The typewriter remained untouched. The drawer beneath the desk stayed locked. Files rested where they belonged. He did not open them. He did not need to. The knowledge that they existed, contained, was enough.

He stood for a moment, listening to the house.

Madhu's breathing upstairs.

The hum of systems functioning quietly.

The distant movement of night insects.

Everything held.

He returned to the bedroom and lay beside Madhu without waking her. Her body adjusted instinctively, moving closer, aligning. Even sleep obeyed the patterns now.

In the days that followed, Madhu's external interactions diminished further.

Not dramatically.

Naturally.

Her parents called, but less often. When they did, Madhu answered with warmth but brevity. She reassured them efficiently, ending conversations before questions could deepen.

Friends no longer reached out at all.

They had accepted the absence.

Absence, Prem knew, required less explanation than refusal.

One afternoon, Madhu sat by the pool and noticed a leaf floating near the edge. She watched it for a long time, curious about why it had not been removed yet. Eventually, a servant appeared silently and lifted it from the water.

Madhu felt relief.

She had not realized the leaf unsettled her.

Later, she mentioned it casually to Prem.

"I don't like when things drift," she said. "It makes me anxious."

Prem nodded. "Uncontained movement creates uncertainty."

She smiled. "I'm glad you notice these things."

"I've always noticed," he replied.

She did not ask what he meant.

That night, during their walk, Madhu slowed near the aviary.

The birds were quieter now, resting. Their colors muted in the low light.

"They don't try to escape anymore," she said softly.

"They never did," Prem replied. "They adjusted."

She accepted that.

The word adjustment no longer sounded temporary.

It sounded complete.

As weeks passed, Madhu's sense of self narrowed further.

She no longer introduced herself by name alone. She introduced herself in relation to Prem, unconsciously mirroring the way others spoke of her. The shift felt subtle, but Prem noticed.

Identity, he knew, did not disappear.

It relocated.

One morning, Madhu woke with a faint sense of unease.

It was unfamiliar enough to disturb her.

She sat up, listening.

The house was quiet.

Too quiet.

She realized the servants were late with breakfast.

The delay unsettled her more than she expected.

She dressed quickly and stepped into the hallway, her steps sharp, purposeful.

A moment later, a servant appeared, apologetic, explaining a minor disruption in the kitchen.

Madhu nodded, reassured instantly.

As soon as order returned, the unease dissolved.

She mentioned the incident to Prem later.

“I felt strange,” she admitted. “Like something was wrong.”

Prem listened carefully. “Routine disruptions can cause discomfort,” he said. “We’ll ensure it doesn’t happen again.”

She relaxed immediately.

That evening, dinner arrived precisely on time.

The next morning, breakfast did too.

Madhu slept better that night.

Prem took note.

Maintenance required vigilance.

Not force.

Precision.

One afternoon, Madhu surprised herself by asking a question she had not allowed in a long time.

"Do you ever think I would have chosen differently," she asked, her tone casual, almost curious.

Prem did not answer immediately.

He chose his words carefully.

"Choice implies awareness of alternatives," he said. "You were always moving toward this life. The rest was noise."

She nodded.

The answer satisfied her.

She did not pursue the thought.

The estate continued its quiet instruction.

Paths subtly redirected foot traffic. Seating encouraged stillness rather than conversation. Lighting softened edges, reducing contrast, reducing friction. Everything worked together to produce the same result.

Calm.

One evening, Madhu stood again near the boundary wall.

The habit resurfaced occasionally, not out of longing, but reflex.

Birds crossed the sky beyond it, fewer now, their movements distant, irrelevant.

Madhu watched briefly, then turned away before Prem joined her.

"I don't feel curious anymore," she said.

"That's good," Prem replied. "Curiosity destabilizes contentment."

She smiled faintly.

They walked back toward the house together, their steps synchronized.

Inside, the estate waited.

Days continued to pass without markers.

No anniversaries were celebrated. No milestones acknowledged. Time did not need to be honored here. It functioned properly on its own.

Madhu's memories of her old life softened further.

She remembered teaching, but without attachment. She remembered friends, but without urgency. She remembered Arjun as one might remember a story heard long ago, its details blurred, its emotional weight neutralized.

Grief, she realized, had not been resolved.

It had been replaced.

One night, she woke suddenly, her heart racing.

For a brief moment, she did not know where she was.

Panic flared.

Then she heard Prem's breathing beside her.

Slow.

Even.

Measured.

The panic dissolved instantly.

She turned toward him, pressing closer, grounding herself in his presence.

In the darkness, she whispered, "I was afraid."

"Of what," Prem asked quietly.

"I don't know," she admitted. "Of being alone."

"You're not," he replied.

She believed him.

The fear did not return.

The following day, Madhu did something she had not done in months.

She tried to imagine leaving.

Not seriously.

Abstractly.

The thought felt uncomfortable almost immediately, like trying to imagine breathing underwater.

Her chest tightened.

Her thoughts scattered.

She stopped the exercise without effort.

Why imagine discomfort.

The estate had taught her not to.

That evening, Prem walked alone through the garden while Madhu slept.

He moved slowly, inspecting nothing, confirming everything. The deer slept. The birds rested. The glass house reflected only darkness and leaves.

Maintenance was complete.

No new inputs were required.

He paused near the boundary wall, placing his hand briefly against the stone.

Solid.

Reliable.

Necessary.

He returned to the house and stood at the doorway to the bedroom, watching Madhu sleep.

Her face was calm.

Untroubled.

Contained.

This, he knew, was the final state.

Not possession.

Not obsession.

Stability.

The most efficient form of control.

Madhu's life no longer required decisions.

Prem's life no longer required effort.

Everything important had been aligned.

Everything unnecessary had been removed.

Maintenance would continue, quietly, indefinitely.

And as long as the systems held, nothing would ever need to change.

Chapter Twenty
The World That Stopped Asking

The first thing Madhu forgot was the sound of urgency.

Not consciously. Not deliberately. It faded the way certain smells fade when one no longer encounters them. She could no longer recall what it felt like to rush toward something undefined, heart slightly elevated, mind racing ahead of her body. The sensation belonged to another version of herself, one she no longer accessed easily.

Inside the estate, nothing hurried.

Time moved, but it did not press. It arranged itself into sequences that required no intervention. Morning followed night. Light softened, then dimmed. Meals appeared. Paths waited. Silence held.

Madhu noticed one morning that she had stopped checking the clock.

The realization came and went without alarm.

She dressed slowly and stepped outside, letting the air decide how long she would stand there. The garden responded as it always did. Leaves stirred gently. Water in the pool lay undisturbed. The deer grazed near the far trees, their movements deliberate, unbothered by observation.

She watched them for a long time.

"They don't look bored," she said later, when Prem joined her.

"They aren't waiting for something else," he replied. "Boredom comes from expectation."

She nodded.

Expectation was something she no longer carried.

Prem's days followed a rhythm that did not require explanation. He left the estate when necessary and returned when it suited the structure he maintained. His absences no longer unsettled Madhu. She trusted that he would return, not because of affection, but because return was part of the design.

Trust, she had learned, did not always come from emotion.

Sometimes it came from predictability.

One afternoon, Madhu walked into a room she had not entered in weeks. It had once held boxes from her earlier life, items she had never unpacked fully. Now the room was empty.

Not cleared hastily.

Resolved.

She stood in the doorway, trying to remember what had been there.

The effort failed.

She did not feel loss.

She felt relief at the simplicity.

That evening, she asked Prem about it.

"I think one of the rooms is empty now," she said casually.

"Yes," he replied. "It wasn't serving a function."

She accepted this easily.

Function had become her preferred measure.

At dinner, conversation remained minimal. Not strained. Complete. They did not need to fill space with commentary. Silence was no longer something to escape. It was something that held.

After dinner, the walk happened as it always did.

Madhu did not think of it as choice. She rose when Prem did. They stepped outside together. The path revealed itself.

They did not go to the glass house that night.

They did not need to.

The entire estate had absorbed its purpose.

As they walked past the deer enclosure, Madhu slowed instinctively.

One deer stood apart from the others, its head raised, eyes focused beyond the fence toward the darkness of the trees.

Madhu followed its gaze.

For a brief moment, she wondered what lay beyond the boundary.

The thought felt unfamiliar.

Uncomfortable.

She turned away.

"They don't leave," she said.

"They don't need to," Prem replied. "Everything they require is here."

She nodded.

Later that night, Madhu woke briefly and listened.

There was no sound of typing.

There had not been for a long time.

The silence did not disturb her.

She no longer needed the reassurance of activity.

The house itself reassured her now.

She returned to sleep without thought.

Days continued to pass.

Madhu's parents stopped asking questions altogether. Their calls were warm but brief, their tone relaxed. They spoke of future visits vaguely, without urgency. Prem handled arrangements. Madhu remained present but uninvolved.

She no longer noticed how little she contributed.

Contribution was not required here.

One afternoon, a distant sound reached the estate from beyond the wall. A siren, faint but unmistakable.

Madhu paused mid-step, her body responding before her mind did.

A flicker of unease passed through her.

She waited.

The sound faded.

The estate returned to quiet.

Her body relaxed instantly.

She did not think about why the sound unsettled her.

She had learned not to investigate discomfort.

That evening, she mentioned it to Prem.

"There was noise earlier," she said. "From outside."

"Yes," he replied. "The city."

"I don't like it," she said.

"You don't have to," he said. "It doesn't belong here."

She felt reassured.

The outside world had begun to feel fictional to her. Something she knew existed, but did not intersect with her life in any meaningful way.

She no longer imagined herself in it.

Her identity had adjusted accordingly.

She was not isolated.

She was contained.

Contained things did not need to engage with what lay beyond their limits.

One morning, Madhu woke with a thought that startled her.

She could not remember the last time she had been alone with her own decisions.

The realization hovered briefly, then dissolved.

Why would she need to remember that.

Choice was not a measure of worth.

The estate had taught her this gently, repeatedly.

Prem noticed her calm deepening.

He had learned long ago that the final stage of control did not look like dominance.

It looked like peace.

No questions. No resistance. No longing.

Just alignment.

That afternoon, he made a small adjustment.

He instructed the staff to change the lighting schedule slightly. Softer in the mornings. Dimmer earlier in the evenings. The shift would reduce contrast, encourage stillness.

Madhu noticed the change and smiled.

"The light feels nicer," she said.

"Yes," Prem replied. "It reduces strain."

She accepted this without reflection.

At night, as they stood on the veranda, Madhu said something quietly, almost to herself.

"I don't think the world needs to know about us."

Prem turned to look at her.

"What do you mean," he asked.

"I mean… we don't need visitors. Or explanations. Or updates," she said. "This is enough."

He studied her for a long moment.

"That's a very clear thought," he said.

She smiled faintly, pleased.

Clarity felt good.

Later, as Madhu slept, Prem walked the estate alone.

He moved along the boundary wall, checking nothing, confirming everything. The stone remained solid. The gate remained closed. Beyond it, distant lights flickered, irrelevant and small.

Inside, the world was complete.

He paused near the glass house.

Its purpose had been fulfilled.

It no longer needed to function as a transition space.

The estate itself was now the cage.

A comfortable one.

An invisible one.

Prem returned to the house and stood outside the bedroom door, listening to Madhu's breathing.

Steady.

Even.

Untroubled.

The world had stopped asking questions.

And so had she.

That, Prem knew, was permanence.

Chapter Twenty-One
The Absence of Want

Want left without ceremony.

It did not announce its departure, did not leave behind a hollow that demanded to be filled. It simply thinned, like a sound heard too often until it blended into background noise and then vanished altogether. Madhu noticed its absence only when she realized she could no longer remember what wanting had once felt like.

She woke one morning with that realization hovering briefly at the edge of her mind.

There was no ache in her chest, no pull toward something unnamed. The day did not present itself as a problem to be solved or a promise to be fulfilled. It was simply there, complete before she touched it.

She lay still, listening to the estate.

The house had its own pulse now, one she recognized instinctively. Pipes murmured softly. The distant hum of systems adjusted temperature and light. Somewhere, a bird shifted within its enclosure. The sound was contained, familiar, unalarming.

Madhu rose and dressed without deliberation.

Her wardrobe no longer represented choice. It represented suitability. Each item existed because it worked within the life she lived. Colors were calm. Textures familiar. Nothing demanded attention.

She stepped outside and walked toward the garden, following a path she did not consciously select. The path selected her.

Morning light fell evenly across the lawn. The deer grazed near the trees, their movements slow and synchronized, as if guided by an unspoken agreement. One lifted its head briefly at her presence, then returned to feeding.

Madhu felt a quiet satisfaction in that recognition.

Prem joined her a few minutes later.

"You're awake early," he said.

"I didn't feel like sleeping longer," she replied. "I felt… finished."

He looked at her carefully, attentive but unalarmed. "Finished how."

"With the day," she said. "Before it started."

He nodded. "That's a sign of stability."

She smiled faintly.

They walked together in silence.

Conversation had become optional now, not because it was discouraged, but because it no longer served a purpose. Words existed to resolve uncertainty. There was no uncertainty left between them.

At breakfast, Madhu noticed she no longer thought about food while eating it. Taste had softened into texture, texture into routine. Eating was no longer an experience. It was a function, performed comfortably.

She did not miss the intensity.

Intensity, she had learned, belonged to imbalance.

Later that morning, she wandered into the study.

This was new.

She had not entered the room freely in a long time. Not because she was forbidden, but because the space did not invite her. It belonged to Prem's earlier life, a place of strategy and construction, of arguments shaped and outcomes decided.

Now, it felt neutral.

The desk stood immaculate. The typewriter rested where it always had, polished, unused, almost ceremonial. The drawers were closed, their contents sealed away in relevance rather than secrecy.

Madhu approached the desk slowly.

She ran her fingers lightly along the edge, then withdrew her hand.

The machine did not interest her.

It had once represented order being created. Now, order existed without effort.

She left the room without looking back.

Outside, the estate adjusted its rhythm around her absence.

Prem watched her from a distance as she crossed the lawn.

She moved differently now.

Not slower.

Contained.

Like someone who no longer needed to scan her environment for possibility or threat.

He had seen this state before.

In animals that had adapted fully to enclosure.

In people who had stopped imagining alternatives.

This was not resignation.

This was acceptance refined into comfort.

In the afternoon, Madhu sat near the pool and watched the water.

She did not think.

She did not reflect.

She allowed the surface to remain undisturbed.

A servant passed quietly and paused.

"Would you like tea," he asked.

Madhu considered the question for a fraction of a second, then nodded.

"Yes."

The answer did not carry preference.

It carried agreement.

When the tea arrived, she drank it slowly, feeling the warmth without evaluating it. Her thoughts did not wander. They did not need to.

She felt no boredom.

Boredom required excess time and insufficient structure.

Here, time was perfectly accounted for.

Later, Prem suggested a drive.

The suggestion surprised her.

She hesitated, feeling a familiar tightening in her chest.

"Do we need to," she asked.

"Only briefly," he replied. "It helps to remember what we're insulated from."

She nodded, trusting him.

The drive was short.

The city appeared briefly at the edges of her vision. Noise pressed against the car. Movement felt erratic. People crossed streets unpredictably, unaware of one another, uncontained.

Madhu felt her shoulders tense.

She did not speak.

Prem noticed and adjusted the route, steering them back toward the estate sooner than planned.

When the gate closed behind them, Madhu exhaled sharply.

"I don't like being out there," she said.

"I know," Prem replied. "You don't belong to disorder."

The phrase settled into her without resistance.

That evening, during their walk, Madhu stopped near the boundary wall.

She rarely did this anymore.

Beyond it, the sky stretched open, darkening into night. A few birds cut across the distance, their silhouettes brief and unanchored.

Madhu watched them without emotion.

"I don't feel anything," she said.

Prem turned to her. "About what."

"About them," she replied. "I used to."

"What did you feel before."

She searched her memory.

"I think I wanted to be like them," she said slowly. "Moving. Unfixed."

"And now."

"I don't understand why," she said. "They look… tired."

Prem nodded. "Movement without purpose exhausts even the strongest."

She turned away from the wall.

The estate received her immediately, its order closing around her like a familiar garment.

That night, Madhu dreamed.

This was unusual now.

In the dream, she stood in the garden alone. The deer watched her from a distance. The birds were silent. The glass house reflected nothing.

She walked toward the gate.

Not with urgency.

With curiosity.

Her hand reached for the latch.

Then she stopped.

In the dream, she realized something.

There was nothing on the other side she needed.

The realization did not frighten her.

It calmed her.

She turned back toward the house.

When she woke, the dream did not linger.

It left behind no residue.

She did not mention it to Prem.

The following days passed without variation.

Madhu no longer measured time by external markers. Days blended seamlessly. Nights followed without drama. There were no events to anticipate, no outcomes to manage.

Her parents called once.

The conversation was brief.

"I just wanted to hear your voice," her mother said.

"I'm fine," Madhu replied. "Everything is calm."

Her mother hesitated. "You sound… distant."

Madhu considered this.

"I feel close to where I am," she said.

Her mother did not know how to respond.

They ended the call politely.

Madhu felt no aftereffect.

The call had not disturbed her equilibrium.

That night, Prem stood beside her in the garden.

"You don't reach outward anymore," he said.

"I don't need to," she replied.

He studied her face carefully.

"Do you ever feel empty," he asked.

She shook her head. "No. I feel… full. But quiet."

He nodded.

Quiet fullness was the most durable state.

As the night deepened, the estate settled into its familiar hush. The deer lay down near the trees. The birds rested within their enclosures. The glass house reflected only shadow and leaves.

Madhu walked back toward the house without waiting for Prem to lead.

Her body knew the way.

Inside the bedroom, she lay down and closed her eyes.

Sleep came quickly.

There was no resistance left.

Prem remained awake a little longer, standing near the window, watching the boundary wall dissolve into darkness.

He did not think about the future.

The future required planning only when instability existed.

Here, everything had reached equilibrium.

Madhu no longer wanted.

And without want, there was no motion.

No questioning.

No escape.

The absence of want was not emptiness.

It was completion.

And completion, once achieved, did not unravel.

It only continued.

Chapter Twenty-Two
The Shape That Remains

The estate did not change when Madhu stopped wanting.

That was the most telling thing.

Nothing responded with alarm or adjustment. No systems recalibrated. No routines shifted. The place did not need to compensate for her internal stillness because it had been designed for it. Want had never been a requirement here. Movement had always been optional. Desire unnecessary.

Madhu sensed this intuitively.

She woke one morning and realized she had not imagined a future in a long time. Not even vaguely. The habit of projecting herself forward had dissolved so quietly that she could not trace when it had ended. There was no anxiety in this realization. Only curiosity, faint and brief.

She sat up in bed and listened.

The house moved gently around her. Pipes murmured. Footsteps passed at measured intervals. Somewhere, a door closed with care. The sounds did not suggest activity so much as confirmation. Everything was where it should be.

She dressed and stepped outside.

The morning air felt exactly as it had the day before. No sharper. No softer. Predictability had become texture. The garden accepted her presence without acknowledgment, as if she were another fixed element rather than a visitor.

The deer stood near the trees, their bodies angled toward the shade. One turned its head slowly and watched her for a moment before returning to grazing. Madhu felt no thrill at being noticed. Recognition no longer mattered.

Prem joined her a few minutes later, his arrival so quiet that she did not hear him until he spoke.

"You're awake," he said.

"I didn't feel like sleeping," she replied.

He nodded. "Sleep responds to need. You're balanced."

The word felt correct.

They walked together without destination.

The paths were familiar enough now that walking them required no attention. Madhu found that her thoughts did not wander during these walks. They did not circle old memories or form new questions. They simply rested, like water held in a basin.

They passed the aviary.

The birds shifted softly, feathers brushing against one another, their movements contained and efficient. Madhu watched them for a while, then moved on.

She no longer compared herself to them.

Comparison required an external reference.

Her world no longer had one.

Later that morning, Madhu sat in a chair near the living room window and watched light move across the floor. She did not follow its progress with interest. She simply allowed it to happen. Time had become something she observed rather than inhabited.

A servant approached quietly and placed a book on the table beside her.

She looked at it without recognition.

“I thought you might like this,” he said.

She nodded politely.

After he left, she opened the book and read a few lines. The language was smooth, the story coherent. She closed it again almost immediately.

Stories felt unnecessary now.

They created tension where none existed.

She did not feel guilty about this.

Guilt belonged to standards she no longer measured herself against.

In the afternoon, Prem left the estate for a short while.

Madhu did not watch him go.

She did not wonder where he went.

She had learned that wondering created a faint ache she did not need.

Instead, she walked toward the boundary wall alone.

This was not a habit she indulged often anymore, but it surfaced occasionally, like a reflex the body had not entirely released.

She stood near the stone and looked outward.

The city lay beyond, distant and indistinct. Sounds reached her only faintly, stripped of urgency by distance and design. A horn sounded somewhere far away, brief and sharp.

Madhu felt nothing.

No irritation.

No longing.

No curiosity.

She placed her hand against the wall and felt its solidity. The stone was cool, unmoving, reliable. The sensation pleased her more than the open space beyond it.

She turned away.

The estate received her again without comment.

When Prem returned, evening had already begun to settle. The light softened, shadows stretched, the garden rearranged itself into night with practiced ease.

They ate dinner together in silence.

Madhu noticed that she no longer evaluated Prem's presence emotionally. She did not ask herself how she felt about him. The relationship had moved beyond feeling. It existed as structure.

Structure did not need validation.

After dinner, they walked as usual.

The night air wrapped around them gently. The trees pressed close, shaping space into corridors that guided their movement without resistance. Madhu followed Prem without thinking. Not because she was directed, but because direction had become unnecessary.

At the glass house, she paused briefly.

She had not been inside it for days.

The structure felt different now.

Not essential.

Historical.

A place that had served a function and then receded into background relevance.

"We don't need to go in," she said.

Prem looked at her carefully. "Do you want to."

She considered the question.

"No," she said. "I don't feel exposed anywhere."

He nodded.

"That means the transition is complete."

She did not ask what he meant.

They continued walking.

That night, Madhu slept without interruption.

No dreams disturbed her. No thoughts lingered at the edge of consciousness. Sleep arrived as function, not escape.

When she woke, she did not remember falling asleep.

Days continued to move in this way.

Madhu's life narrowed further, but without tension. Narrowing had once suggested loss to her. Now it suggested focus. The removal of excess.

She did not miss her old routines.

She did not miss her work.

She did not miss her friends.

Missing required absence.

Everything she needed was present.

One afternoon, a letter arrived.

It was addressed to Madhu in handwriting she recognized only after a moment's effort. An old colleague. A teacher she had once worked closely with. The letter was polite, concerned, curious.

Madhu read it slowly.

It asked how she was.

It mentioned the past.

It suggested meeting.

Madhu folded the letter carefully and placed it back in the envelope.

She did not feel compelled to respond.

The letter did not anger her.

It simply felt irrelevant.

When Prem found it later on the table, he did not comment. He picked it up, placed it in a drawer, and closed it.

The action felt like maintenance.

Madhu felt relief.

That evening, as they walked, Madhu said something quietly.

"I think I'm finished becoming."

Prem turned to her.

"What do you mean," he asked.

"I don't feel like there's another version of me waiting," she said. "I think this is it."

He studied her face carefully, searching for uncertainty.

He found none.

"That's a rare state," he said. "Most people never reach it."

She smiled faintly.

"I don't feel rare," she said. "I feel ordinary."

"That's the highest form of stability," he replied.

They walked on.

Later that night, Prem stood alone near the boundary wall.

He had begun doing this more often.

Not because he felt drawn to what lay beyond it, but because confirming the boundary reassured him. The wall existed. The gate remained closed. The systems held.

Beyond the estate, the world continued its unpredictable motion.

Inside, nothing shifted.

He returned to the house and paused outside the bedroom door.

Madhu slept peacefully.

Her breathing was steady.

He listened for a moment longer than necessary, then entered quietly and lay beside her.

Her body adjusted instinctively, aligning without waking.

Even sleep obeyed the structure now.

The next morning, Madhu woke with a thought that felt almost foreign.

She wondered what day it was.

The question lingered briefly, then dissolved.

The answer did not matter.

She dressed and stepped outside.

The garden greeted her as it always did.

The deer grazed.

The birds moved within their limits.

The house waited.

Madhu moved through her life without friction.

She no longer sought meaning.

Meaning required distance.

Here, there was only presence.

The shape of her life had settled into something smooth, continuous, and unbroken.

There were no edges left to catch on.

No questions left to ask.

And as the days continued to pass without distinction, the estate held her gently within its design.

The shape that remained did not ask to be altered.

It simply endured.

Chapter Twenty Three
What Persists

Change arrived so quietly that Madhu did not recognize it as change.

It did not come as disruption or demand. It came as an adjustment so small it felt like nothing at all. A fraction of light altered. A sound softened. A pause lengthened. The estate absorbed it before she could form a thought about it.

She woke one morning and realized she had not spoken aloud in a long time.

The realization did not alarm her.

Speech, she understood, was a tool. Tools were used when needed. Here, nothing required explanation. The house already knew how to respond.

She dressed and stepped outside.

The morning air felt balanced. Neither cool nor warm. The garden held stillness the way water holds reflection. The deer grazed at a measured distance, their bodies relaxed, their movements efficient.

Madhu watched them without emotion.

She did not feel affection.

She did not feel envy.

She felt recognition.

Prem joined her a few moments later.

"You are quiet," he said.

"I do not feel unfinished," she replied.

He nodded.

That was enough.

They walked together without choosing a path. The path formed naturally beneath their steps. Trees framed their movement. Light guided them forward. The estate did not present options. It presented continuity.

Later that morning, Madhu sat in a chair by the living room window.

She did not read.

She did not think.

She watched light move.

Time passed without texture.

At some point, a servant placed a glass of water beside her. She drank it when her body signaled thirst. Not desire. Need.

Her mind did not wander.

This absence of wandering had become normal.

Prem watched her from the doorway.

He noted the stillness in her posture. The lack of micro movement that once accompanied thought. The way her breathing had synchronized with the house itself.

He had seen this state before.

In people who had stopped negotiating with themselves.

At midday, Prem left the estate.

Madhu did not register his departure.

She no longer marked absence.

Absence implied return. Return implied waiting.

She did neither.

Instead, she walked toward the boundary wall.

This had become an occasional movement. Not curiosity. Habit.

She placed her hand on the stone and felt its texture.

Solid.

Unyielding.

She closed her eyes briefly and stood there.

There was no image in her mind.

No memory.

No future.

Just pressure against skin.

She opened her eyes and turned away.

The estate accepted her again.

When Prem returned in the late afternoon, Madhu was sitting near the pool.

The water lay perfectly still.

He sat beside her without speaking.

They did not touch.

Touch had become unnecessary to confirm presence.

After a while, Madhu said something quietly.

"I think I would disappear if this place disappeared."

Prem turned slightly toward her.

"Places shape people," he said. "This one shapes you correctly."

She nodded.

There was no fear in her statement.

Only fact.

That evening, the estate adjusted again.

Lights dimmed earlier than usual. Paths softened into shadow. The night arrived without edge.

They walked.

The deer were already still.

The birds were quiet.

The glass house reflected nothing but trees and darkness.

Madhu did not glance at it.

It had completed its role.

Inside the house later, Madhu noticed something missing.

She could not name it.

The sensation hovered briefly, then resolved.

She did not pursue it.

Prem noticed her pause.

"What is it," he asked.

"I thought something was supposed to be here," she said. "But I cannot remember what."

He considered this carefully.

"Then it was unnecessary," he replied.

She accepted this instantly.

That night, Madhu slept without dreaming.

When she woke, she did not know how long she had slept.

The distinction no longer mattered.

Days followed.

The estate continued its rhythm.

Madhu no longer counted time in days.

She counted it in repetitions.

Walk.

Sit.

Eat.

Sleep.

Each cycle identical.

Each cycle reassuring.

One afternoon, a sound reached the estate that had not arrived in months.

Laughter.

Distant.

Human.

From beyond the wall.

Madhu paused.

The sound struck something dormant inside her.

Not emotion.

Recognition.

She turned toward the sound instinctively.

Her body tensed slightly.

The sound faded.

Silence returned.

Madhu exhaled.

The tension dissolved.

She did not analyze the reaction.

Analysis created friction.

That evening, she mentioned it to Prem.

"There was laughter outside," she said.

"Yes," he replied. "Occasionally the world leaks."

"I did not like it," she said.

"That is because it does not belong to you," he replied.

She nodded.

The statement settled easily.

Prem did not miss what Madhu had lost.

Loss was irrelevant.

He measured success by absence of resistance.

And there was none.

Madhu moved through the estate as if she had been born within its walls.

Her posture reflected certainty.

Her gaze no longer searched.

She no longer mirrored others.

She no longer reacted.

She existed.

One night, as Prem stood near the boundary wall alone, he noticed something new.

The city lights beyond the estate seemed dimmer.

Not because they had changed.

Because they no longer registered.

He placed his hand against the stone.

The boundary felt permanent.

As it should.

Inside the house, Madhu slept peacefully.

Her face was smooth.

Untroubled.

He watched her for a moment, then turned away.

The system was complete.

Nothing required adjustment.

Nothing required correction.

Only repetition.

Madhu woke the next morning and did not remember her name immediately.

The thought arrived later, without urgency.

Madhu.

The name did not carry identity.

It functioned as a label.

She accepted it and moved on.

She stepped outside.

The garden waited.

The deer grazed.

The birds moved within their limits.

The house held its shape.

Madhu moved through her life without reflection.

There were no edges left.

No friction.

No hunger.

No future.

Only continuation.

And continuation, when perfected, no longer needed awareness.

It simply persisted.

Chapter Twenty Four
The Return of a Question

The question arrived without sound.

It did not announce itself the way questions used to, sharp and insistent, demanding answers. It slipped into Madhu's mind like a ripple that barely disturbed the surface, subtle enough to be mistaken for a passing sensation.

She noticed it while standing in the garden.

The deer grazed near the trees, their movements steady, their bodies relaxed. The air held the mild warmth of late afternoon. Nothing in the environment suggested interruption.

And yet, something stirred.

Madhu watched one deer lift its head and pause. Its ears angled slightly, responding to something beyond her perception. The animal did not run. It did not tense. It simply listened, then returned to grazing.

The motion stayed with her.

Not as emotion.

As pattern.

She realized she was listening too.

Not for sound.

For difference.

The sensation passed quickly, but it left a faint trace, like a footprint in soft earth. Madhu did not pursue it. Pursuit implied intention. Intention implied dissatisfaction.

She had neither.

Prem joined her moments later.

"You've been standing here a long time," he said.

"I didn't notice," she replied.

He studied her face, attentive without concern. "You look thoughtful."

"I don't feel anything," she said. "I was just… still."

He nodded. Stillness was not new. It was their shared language now.

They walked together toward the house.

Inside, the estate maintained its rhythm. Light adjusted. Doors closed softly. The quiet remained intact.

Madhu sat in the living room and watched shadows shift across the floor. Time passed without pressure. The house absorbed it effortlessly.

And yet, the trace remained.

Later that evening, as they ate dinner, Madhu found herself pausing between bites.

The pause was unfamiliar.

Prem noticed.

"Is something wrong," he asked calmly.

"No," she replied immediately. "I think I was distracted."

"By what."

She searched her mind and found no object. "Nothing."

He accepted this.

But he noted the hesitation.

That night, Madhu slept.

Her dreams returned.

This alone was unusual.

In the dream, she stood in the glass house. The trees pressed close, their shapes reflected endlessly in the transparent walls. She could see herself from multiple angles, each reflection slightly delayed, slightly altered.

She reached out to touch the glass.

Her reflection did not respond.

Behind her, the estate stretched outward, vast and ordered. Ahead of her, beyond the glass, there was no visible boundary, only darkness and movement she could not name.

A sound emerged.

Not a voice.

A question without words.

She woke abruptly.

Her heart beat faster than usual.

The room was dark. The house quiet. Prem's breathing beside her steady and even.

The familiarity grounded her immediately.

She lay still until her pulse slowed.

In the morning, she did not mention the dream.

Dreams, she had learned, were remnants of imbalance.

They faded when ignored.

The day resumed its pattern.

Walks. Silence. Routine.

But the trace did not disappear.

It surfaced again in small, unexpected ways.

When a servant adjusted a vase slightly off-center, Madhu noticed before the correction was made. The brief misalignment unsettled her more than she expected. Relief followed when order returned.

She did not comment.

When the lighting dimmed earlier than usual one evening, she felt a flicker of irritation, then calm once it stabilized.

These reactions were subtle.

But new.

Prem observed them quietly.

Not with alarm.

With interest.

That afternoon, Prem left the estate for longer than usual.

Madhu noticed his absence this time.

Not as anxiety.

As awareness.

She sat by the pool and watched the water. A faint breeze disturbed the surface briefly, creating ripples that took longer than usual to settle.

She found herself waiting.

For the water to become still again.

When it did, her shoulders relaxed.

She realized then that she had been holding tension.

The realization startled her.

She had not held tension in a long time.

The trace sharpened.

By the time Prem returned, dusk had settled.

Madhu was standing near the boundary wall.

She did not remember walking there.

She was simply there.

The city beyond remained distant, indistinct, but a faint sound drifted over the stone. Traffic. Voices. Movement.

The sound did not frighten her.

It irritated her.

Prem approached quietly.

“You’re close to the wall,” he said.

“Yes,” she replied. “I didn’t mean to come here.”

He joined her, placing himself between her and the boundary without making it obvious.

“Is something bothering you,” he asked.

She hesitated.

Hesitation itself felt unfamiliar.

“I don’t know,” she said. “I keep noticing things.”

“What kind of things.”

“When things change,” she replied. “Even a little.”

He considered this carefully.

“Change can feel disruptive when life is stable,” he said. “It doesn’t mean anything is wrong.”

She nodded.

His explanation soothed her.

Still, the trace remained.

That night, the dream returned.

This time, she stood at the gate.

Her hand rested on the metal latch.

She did not feel fear.

She did not feel desire.

She felt curiosity.

The gate did not open.

She woke before anything happened.

The next morning, Madhu found herself looking for the glass house.

She had not thought about it consciously in weeks.

She walked toward it alone.

The structure stood unchanged, its surfaces reflecting trees and sky. It felt distant now, like a place she had once needed but no longer did.

She stepped inside.

The air felt different.

Not warmer.

Not cooler.

Empty.

She stood there for a long moment.

Nothing happened.

The glass reflected her image clearly.

She studied herself.

Her face was calm.

Her posture relaxed.

But something in her eyes felt unfamiliar.

Not longing.

Not fear.

Recognition.

She left the glass house and returned to the main path.

By the time Prem joined her later, the moment had already dulled.

Still, he sensed something.

"You went to the glass house," he said.

"Yes," she replied. "I wanted to see if it felt the same."

"And did it."

"No," she said. "It felt finished."

He nodded. "That's normal. It served its purpose."

"What purpose," she asked.

The question landed lightly.

But it landed.

Prem answered without pause. "Transition."

She accepted this.

Yet the word echoed faintly in her mind long after the conversation ended.

Transition implied before and after.

She had not thought in those terms for a long time.

That evening, as they walked, Madhu slowed unexpectedly.

"Prem," she said.

"Yes."

"Do you remember when we first walked here together."

He considered the question carefully.

"Yes."

She frowned slightly. "I don't."

He watched her closely.

"That's not unusual," he said. "Early memories fade when they're no longer relevant."

She nodded.

The explanation satisfied her.

But the question lingered, quiet and unresolved.

That night, Prem stood alone in the study for the first time in months.

He did not open the drawer.

He did not touch the typewriter.

He simply stood and listened to the house.

Madhu's breathing upstairs.

The hum of systems.

The silence.

Everything held.

And yet, something had shifted.

Not broken.

Shifted.

Prem understood this.

Systems did not fail abruptly.

They developed micro fractures.

Not dangerous.

Informative.

He returned to the bedroom and lay beside Madhu.

She adjusted instinctively, moving closer.

Her body still obeyed the structure.

That reassured him.

The next morning, Madhu woke with the faintest sense of anticipation.

She did not know why.

She did not name it.

She simply noticed it.

As she dressed, she paused in front of the mirror.

For the first time in a long while, she studied her reflection.

Not critically.

Curiously.

She touched her own face lightly, as if confirming it was still there.

It was.

She smiled faintly and stepped away.

Outside, the garden waited.

The deer grazed.

The birds moved within their limits.

The estate remained unchanged.

And yet, somewhere beneath the calm, a question had returned.

It did not ask to be answered.

Not yet.

It simply existed.

Waiting.

CHAPTER TWENTY FIVE
CONTAINMENT TESTED

The disturbance did not arrive through the gate.

It came through the calendar.

Madhu noticed it when Prem mentioned the date casually, as if he were noting the weather or the time of day.

"There's a function next week," he said one evening, as they sat in the living room after dinner. "A legal conclave. Two days. Out of town."

Madhu looked up.

Not sharply.

Just enough.

"Oh," she said.

The sound left her mouth before thought followed it.

Prem observed the reaction carefully. It was subtle, but it existed. A pause. A shift in posture. A momentary recalibration of attention.

"You don't have to come," he added immediately, his tone neutral. "It's not necessary."

The word unnecessary usually settled Madhu.

This time, it hovered.

"I could," she said.

The sentence surprised both of them.

Prem did not show it.

"You could," he agreed. "If you want."

Want.

The word felt strange in her mouth, like a language she no longer spoke fluently.

She nodded once. "I think I should."

Should was easier.

Prem leaned back slightly, studying her face without appearing to.

"Travel disrupts routine," he said. "It can be tiring."

"I'll be with you," she replied.

The logic sounded complete.

He nodded. "We'll see."

The conversation ended there.

But something had been introduced.

Not conflict.

Context.

That night, Madhu slept lightly.

Not restlessly.

Just less deeply.

Dreams did not come, but awareness lingered near the surface. She woke once, then again, listening to the house.

Everything was normal.

That unsettled her.

In the morning, she noticed small things more acutely than usual.

The way the servants spoke to one another in low voices near the kitchen. The faint sound of a vehicle passing beyond the boundary wall. A bird calling from outside the estate, its sound unfamiliar.

None of these things were new.

But today, she noticed them.

She did not comment.

She walked the garden longer than usual, circling paths that usually satisfied her quickly. When she reached the deer enclosure, she stopped and watched them carefully.

One deer moved closer to the fence than the others, its head raised, ears alert. It stood that way for several seconds before retreating slowly back into the group.

Madhu felt something tighten in her chest.

Not fear.

Recognition.

She mirrored the movement unconsciously, stepping closer to the fence, then stopping.

She did not know why she had moved at all.

Later that day, Prem left the estate to attend a meeting.

Madhu noticed his absence immediately.

This was new.

She did not feel anxious.

She felt… unanchored.

The feeling irritated her more than frightened her.

She sat by the pool, then stood, then walked inside, then returned to the garden. The movements lacked purpose. She recognized this as inefficiency.

She did not like inefficiency.

When Prem returned that evening, she was standing near the glass house.

He approached quietly.

"You went there today," he said.

"Yes," she replied. "I didn't go inside."

He nodded. "Did it feel different."

"Yes," she said honestly. "It felt like a place that belongs to the past."

"That's because it does," Prem replied.

She accepted this.

Still, she remained near the structure longer than usual, as if waiting for it to say something.

It did not.

That night, Madhu asked a question she had not planned to ask.

"What happens when we leave the estate for two days," she said.

Prem did not answer immediately.

The pause was deliberate.

"The estate remains," he said. "Structure doesn't dissolve when you step away from it."

She nodded, reassured.

But the reassurance was intellectual.

Not embodied.

The next day, preparations began.

Not for travel.

For insulation.

Prem did not announce this.

He never did.

But Madhu noticed subtle changes.

The staff schedule adjusted. Lights were tested at different hours. Supplies were restocked more thoroughly than usual. Paths were cleared with extra precision.

The estate was being prepared to function without them.

This realization unsettled her.

Not because she feared absence.

Because the estate did not seem to need her.

That evening, her parents called.

This was unusual.

They rarely called without prior arrangement now.

Madhu answered after a brief hesitation.

“We heard you might be traveling,” her mother said.

Madhu frowned. “How did you know.”

“Prem mentioned it,” her father replied. “He thought we should be informed.”

Madhu felt a flicker of irritation.

Not at her parents.

At the idea of information moving without her.

“Yes,” she said. “Just for a couple of days.”

Her mother hesitated. “Would you like to stay with us afterward. Even for one night.”

The suggestion landed harder than expected.

Madhu opened her mouth to respond, then stopped.

She felt heat rise in her chest.

Not anger.

Pressure.

“I don’t think so,” she said quickly. “That would be too much movement.”

Her mother was silent for a moment.

“You sound tense,” she said gently.

"I'm not," Madhu replied. "I just don't like disruption."

After the call ended, Madhu sat very still.

She placed her phone on the table and stared at it, as if it were an object she did not fully recognize.

Prem entered the room a few minutes later.

"You handled that well," he said.

Madhu looked up sharply.

"Well," she repeated.

"Yes," he said. "You protected your stability."

The word stabilized her.

She nodded.

Still, that night, she dreamed again.

In the dream, she stood inside the estate while everything else moved.

The house shifted slightly, as if floating. The paths rearranged. The deer moved restlessly. The birds fluttered against their enclosures.

Madhu stood still, unable to move.

The estate did not respond to her presence.

She woke with her heart beating faster than usual.

The morning came.

Preparations continued.

Madhu began to feel something unfamiliar.

Anticipation.

Not excitement.

Readiness.

The day before departure, Prem walked her through the estate.

Not overtly.

Subtly.

They walked each familiar path. Passed each structure. Paused briefly at the deer enclosure.

"They will be fine," Prem said, as if answering an unspoken concern.

Madhu nodded.

She realized then that she was thinking about what would happen in her absence.

This disturbed her.

The estate was not supposed to require her consideration.

That evening, she stood near the boundary wall longer than she had in months.

The city beyond was audible now. Not loud. Present.

Movement existed there.

Unstructured.

Madhu felt irritation rise again.

"I don't like knowing it's there," she said when Prem joined her.

"It doesn't concern you," he replied.

She nodded.

But she did not step away immediately.

That night, Prem returned to the study.

This, too, was new.

He did not turn on the main light.

He did not open the drawer.

He simply stood there for a long time, listening.

Systems responded well under pressure.

But travel introduced variables.

Variables required attention.

Madhu slept fitfully.

In the morning, she dressed carefully.

Too carefully.

Prem noticed.

"You're overthinking," he said.

"Yes," she replied. "I don't like that."

They drove out of the estate late morning.

The gate opened.

The moment stretched longer than usual.

Madhu watched the boundary wall recede.

Her chest tightened.

Not fear.

Loss of reference.

The city pressed in almost immediately.

Noise.

Movement.

People.

Madhu stiffened in her seat.

Prem drove calmly.

"We'll return soon," he said.

She nodded, clinging to the promise.

At the hotel, Madhu felt exposed.

The walls felt thin.

The silence felt wrong.

She did not unpack fully.

She sat on the bed and waited.

For what, she did not know.

That evening, they attended the event.

People spoke.

Too much.

They looked at her.

Asked questions.

She answered mechanically.

Her head began to ache.

When they returned to the room, Madhu removed her shoes and sat on the floor.

"I don't like being here," she said flatly.

Prem crouched beside her.

"I know," he said. "This is temporary."

She looked at him.

Her eyes searched his face for something she had not needed in a long time.

Reassurance.

Not explanation.

"Promise we'll go back tomorrow," she said.

"Yes," he replied without hesitation.

That night, Madhu did not sleep.

The city did not quiet itself the way the estate did.

Sounds leaked through walls.

Doors opened and closed unpredictably.

A siren passed in the distance.

Madhu covered her ears briefly, then lowered her hands, embarrassed by the impulse.

She lay awake, staring at the ceiling.

For the first time in months, she thought clearly.

This place does not hold me.

The thought frightened her.

When morning arrived, she felt relief.

Not because of the day.

Because they would leave.

On the drive back, Madhu said very little.

When the estate gate finally closed behind them, she exhaled sharply, as if she had been holding her breath for hours.

She leaned back in her seat.

"I don't want to leave again," she said.

"You won't have to," Prem replied.

Inside the estate, the air felt heavier.

Warmer.

More complete.

Madhu stepped out of the car and stood still.

Her body relaxed instantly.

She did not realize how tense she had been until now.

That evening, as they walked the garden, Madhu felt something settle firmly into place.

The disturbance had been tested.

It had failed.

The estate had reasserted itself.

Later that night, Madhu slept deeply.

No dreams.

No questions.

Prem stood alone near the boundary wall, listening to the city fade into irrelevance once more.

Containment had been tested.

Containment had held.

Nothing further would challenge it.

Not now.

Not ever.

Chapter Twenty Six
The Perfect Cage

The morning after their return did not feel like a return at all.

Madhu woke before the light fully entered the room, her body already aligned with the estate's rhythm. The unfamiliar weight she had carried during the journey was gone. Her breath moved easily. Her limbs rested without tension. The ceiling above her felt neither high nor low. It was simply correct.

She lay still for a moment, listening.

The house answered her in the language she now understood best. Pipes murmured softly. A door closed at the far end with careful restraint. Footsteps passed, measured and familiar. Somewhere, water began to run, then stopped.

Everything was back where it belonged.

Madhu sat up and felt relief settle into her bones.

She dressed without thought, choosing clothes that did not announce themselves. The fabric rested against her skin without friction. She stepped outside and let the air confirm what she already knew.

The estate had not changed.

The garden lay in its usual balance, trimmed and contained, paths guiding the eye as much as the feet. The pool reflected the sky with perfect indifference. The deer grazed near the trees, their bodies relaxed, their movements efficient.

Madhu watched them for a long time.

Not with affection.

With understanding.

Prem joined her silently.

"You slept," he said.

"Yes," she replied. "Immediately."

He nodded. "Your body recognizes where it belongs."

She did not question the statement.

They walked together, their steps naturally synchronized. The path did not require decision. It revealed itself.

They passed the deer enclosure. One animal lifted its head briefly, then lowered it again, unbothered by their presence. Madhu felt no impulse to stop.

She no longer needed to measure herself against them.

They continued walking until the house reabsorbed them.

Inside, breakfast waited.

Madhu ate slowly, noticing that the food tasted familiar again. The mildness that had comforted her for months returned fully. She realized then how sharp and intrusive flavors had felt during the trip, how the city had insisted on being experienced.

Here, nothing insisted.

Prem watched her with quiet satisfaction.

He did not need to ask how she felt.

Her posture answered him.

The day unfolded with deliberate simplicity.

Madhu did not wander restlessly. She did not seek distraction. She moved from one space to another with purpose, even when the purpose was simply to sit and exist.

She returned briefly to the glass house.

Not because she felt drawn to it.

Because she wanted to confirm something.

Inside, the structure felt neutral. The glass reflected trees and sky without distortion. The space no longer held tension or promise.

She stood there and realized the truth with calm certainty.

The glass house was no longer the cage.

It had been a lesson.

She stepped out and did not look back.

That afternoon, Prem returned to his study.

This time, he did sit at the desk.

He did not open files.

He did not type.

He simply sat, the presence of the room reasserting itself around him.

The machine remained silent.

Silence was now the preferred state.

Madhu did not enter the study.

She did not feel excluded.

She felt unnecessary to the function occurring there.

That was comforting.

In the late afternoon, Madhu stood near the boundary wall again.

The habit had not entirely vanished.

But the impulse felt different now.

She stood there not to look beyond, but to confirm the boundary's existence.

The city beyond was audible in faint fragments. A horn. A distant voice. A movement that did not resolve into pattern.

Madhu felt irritation rise and then pass.

She placed her palm against the stone.

The solidity pleased her.

She turned away without hesitation.

That evening, Prem suggested they skip the walk.

This, too, was new.

Madhu nodded without question.

Skipping no longer felt like deviation.

It felt like refinement.

They stayed inside.

The house adjusted, drawing inward, light softening earlier than usual. The estate did not require ritual to function. It required only alignment.

Madhu sat near the window and watched the darkness gather.

"I don't want to go out again," she said quietly.

Prem did not pretend to misunderstand.

"You won't," he replied.

The simplicity of the promise settled something permanently inside her.

That night, Madhu slept deeply.

There were no dreams.

Not even fragments.

When she woke, she did not remember falling asleep.

Days followed.

They were identical.

Not monotonous.

Complete.

Madhu stopped marking them entirely.

She woke. She moved. She ate. She rested. She slept.

Each action flowed into the next without friction.

Her parents called once.

The conversation was brief.

They spoke of ordinary things. Weather. Health. Distant relatives.

Madhu answered politely, efficiently.

When the call ended, she did not feel the echo of voices lingering in her head.

The house absorbed the silence immediately.

Friends no longer reached out at all.

The absence felt correct.

Absence, she had learned, was not loss when there was no space left to fill.

One afternoon, Madhu found an old notebook while a drawer was being reorganized.

It contained her handwriting.

Questions.

Annotations.

Arguments.

She flipped through it without recognition.

The words felt excessive.

She closed the notebook and handed it to a servant.

"Store this," she said.

The servant nodded and removed it.

Madhu felt lighter.

She did not wonder where it would go.

That night, Prem walked the estate alone.

He did this occasionally now, not to check, but to confirm.

The deer slept near the tree line.

The birds rested within their enclosures.

The glass house reflected nothing but shadow.

The boundary wall held firm.

Everything was in place.

He returned to the house and paused outside the bedroom.

Madhu slept peacefully.

Her breathing was steady.

Untroubled.

He lay beside her.

Her body adjusted instinctively, aligning without waking.

Even sleep obeyed the design now.

The following morning, Madhu woke with no trace of the city left in her memory.

The trip already felt abstract, like a story someone else had told her.

She stood before the mirror briefly.

Her reflection did not ask questions.

Her face carried no conflict.

She stepped away.

Outside, the estate waited.

She walked the garden alone, passing each familiar marker without stopping.

The pool.

The paths.

The trees.

She paused near the deer enclosure only once.

One deer stood close to the fence, its body relaxed, eyes half-lidded.

Madhu looked at it and felt a quiet certainty settle fully into place.

It does not know it is contained.

It does not need to.

The thought did not frighten her.

It reassured her.

Later that day, Prem suggested a minor adjustment.

"We'll move dinner earlier," he said. "It suits the light better."

Madhu nodded. "That's better."

There was no discussion.

The change took effect immediately.

She felt no disruption.

That night, she noticed something important.

She did not think about thinking.

The internal commentary that once narrated her life was gone.

Silence had moved inside her.

Not emptiness.

Stillness.

Prem recognized this too.

This was the final stage.

Not obedience.

Not dependence.

Integration.

The system no longer required reinforcement.

Madhu had internalized the structure completely.

There were no questions left to neutralize.

No curiosity left to redirect.

No memory strong enough to disturb equilibrium.

The cage no longer needed bars.

It had become perspective.

Late that night, Madhu stirred briefly.

Not waking fully.

She whispered something unintelligible, then settled again.

Prem listened.

He did not need to understand the words.

Meaning no longer mattered.

Only continuation.

Morning arrived.

The estate woke.

Madhu moved through her day without effort.

Nothing pressed against her.

Nothing pulled her outward.

Nothing asked to be changed.

She lived entirely within the shape provided to her.

The perfect cage did not announce itself.

It did not hurt.

It did not restrict.

It did not feel like confinement at all.

It felt like peace.

And peace, once perfected, required no escape.

It only required time.

Chapter Twenty Seven
Nothing Left to Open

Morning arrived without announcement.

Madhu woke before light reached the far corners of the room, not because something stirred inside her, but because waking had become part of the estate's rhythm. Her eyes opened easily. Her body did not hesitate. There was no moment of orientation, no question of where she was.

She was here.

That was enough.

She lay still for a short while, listening. The house spoke softly around her, a language of structure she no longer translated into thought. Pipes murmured. Footsteps passed at a respectful distance. Somewhere, a door closed with precision.

Nothing improvised.

Nothing accidental.

She rose, dressed, and stepped outside.

The garden held its shape perfectly. Dew clung to leaves in the same places it always did. The paths curved gently, guiding her forward without asking where she wished to go. The pool reflected the sky, smooth and undisturbed.

The deer grazed near the trees.

Madhu watched them without stopping.

She did not feel drawn to them anymore. She did not seek meaning in their presence. They were simply part of the estate's composition, like the trees or the walls or the light.

Prem joined her moments later.

"You're awake early," he said.

"Yes," she replied.

There was no reason given.

There was no reason required.

They walked together in silence. Not the silence of restraint, but the silence of completion. Words would have introduced unnecessary variation.

As they passed the deer enclosure, one animal lifted its head briefly and then lowered it again. Madhu did not slow her steps.

She no longer needed mirrors.

They returned to the house.

Breakfast appeared.

Madhu ate without attention, not because the food lacked taste, but because taste no longer required evaluation. Eating was not pleasure or discipline. It was maintenance.

She noticed, distantly, that she no longer remembered what foods she used to like or dislike.

Preference had dissolved.

Later that morning, Prem left for his study.

He did not tell her.

He did not need to.

Madhu did not track his movement. She did not wait for his return. Waiting belonged to anticipation, and anticipation belonged to a life that expected change.

She sat near the living room window and watched light move across the floor.

Time passed.

She did not count it.

At some point, a servant adjusted the curtains slightly, refining the angle of light. Madhu felt relief without knowing why.

Order restored itself automatically.

She closed her eyes briefly.

Nothing surfaced.

No memories pressed forward.

No images demanded attention.

Her mind rested the way water rests when undisturbed.

In the afternoon, she walked toward the glass house.

Not deliberately.

It appeared in her path, and she acknowledged it.

She stood outside it for a moment, studying the reflection. Trees, sky, her own outline, all layered without hierarchy.

She stepped inside.

The space felt empty of meaning.

Not cold.

Not warm.

Finished.

She stood there and felt no emotion.

No memory.

No attachment.

The glass house did not speak to her anymore.

It had already said everything it needed to say.

She stepped back out and continued walking, leaving it behind without ceremony.

That evening, Prem returned from the study.

He looked at Madhu carefully.

"You went to the glass house," he said.

"Yes," she replied.

"And."

"There was nothing there," she said calmly.

He nodded.

That was the correct answer.

They did not walk that night.

They did not need to.

The house itself had absorbed the ritual.

As darkness settled, the estate drew inward, light softening, shadows aligning into familiar shapes. The boundary wall stood firm, invisible from inside unless sought.

Madhu did not seek it.

She sat beside Prem in the living room, her posture relaxed, her presence steady.

After a long while, she spoke.

"I don't think about before anymore," she said.

Prem turned slightly toward her.

"Does that bother you."

She considered the question seriously.

"No," she said. "It feels efficient."

Efficiency.

The word settled into the space between them like a final seal.

That night, Madhu slept deeply.

There were no dreams.

Not even fragments.

When she woke, she did not know how long she had slept, and the thought did not trouble her.

Days passed.

They were indistinguishable.

Madhu no longer noticed the passing.

She did not mark weeks or months.

Her parents called once more.

The conversation was short.

They spoke of health, of routine, of ordinary things that required no emotional response.

Madhu answered politely.

When the call ended, she placed the phone down and did not think of it again.

The device did not pull at her attention.

Attention belonged to systems, not objects.

One afternoon, Madhu stood near the boundary wall.

The habit had not disappeared entirely, but its meaning had changed.

She stood there not to look beyond, but to feel the stone beneath her palm.

Solid.

Defined.

Necessary.

Beyond it, the city made noise.

Movement.

Uncontained sound.

Madhu felt irritation rise and then fade.

She turned away without hesitation.

The estate received her immediately.

That night, Prem walked alone through the garden.

He did this now without intention, not to inspect, not to correct.

Only to confirm.

The deer lay still near the trees.

The birds rested within their enclosures.

The glass house reflected nothing but darkness and leaves.

Everything remained.

Nothing shifted.

He stopped near the boundary wall and placed his hand against the stone.

It did not move.

It never would.

Inside the house, Madhu slept peacefully.

Her face was calm.

Untroubled.

He watched her for a moment before lying down beside her.

Her body adjusted instinctively, aligning without waking.

Even unconsciousness obeyed the design.

Morning returned.

Madhu rose.

She dressed.

She stepped outside.

The garden waited.

She walked its paths without thought.

She did not feel watched.

She did not feel confined.

She did not feel protected.

She simply felt correct.

At the deer enclosure, one animal stood close to the fence, its body relaxed, eyes half-lidded.

Madhu paused briefly.

Not to observe.

To acknowledge.

It did not know it was contained.

It did not need to.

She turned and walked back toward the house.

Inside, Prem stood near the window, watching the light shift across the floor.

He did not turn when she entered.

He knew she was there.

Presence no longer required confirmation.

Madhu stood beside him.

For a long moment, neither spoke.

Then Madhu said something quietly.

"I don't think there's anywhere else for me."

Prem did not smile.

He did not reassure.

He did not respond emotionally.

He simply said, "There never was."

The words did not land as revelation.

They landed as fact.

Outside, the estate held its shape.

Inside, Madhu lived without edges.

No questions returned.

No doors appeared.

No truth emerged.

Nothing opened.

And nothing ever would.

Chapter Twenty Eight
Years, Unmarked

Time did not announce itself with anniversaries.

It moved through the estate the way weather did, adjusting light, softening stone, deepening shadows without asking to be acknowledged. Seasons passed not as events but as calibrations. Leaves fell where they were expected to fall. Grass returned where it had been trimmed. The paths remained obedient to their curves.

Madhu did not count the years.

She had stopped counting days long before that.

Morning arrived and she woke. Evening arrived and she rested. Night came and she slept. Between those points, life happened without urgency, without variation that demanded attention.

If someone had asked her how long she had lived here, she would not have known how to answer.

The estate did not measure time the way the outside world did.

It measured stability.

Madhu moved through her days with the same ease she once reserved for sleep. She dressed, walked, ate, rested. Her body followed routines that no longer felt imposed. They felt instinctive, as if her muscles had learned the layout of the place and now responded to it automatically.

She did not think of this as discipline.

She thought of it as alignment.

Prem's presence remained constant.

He left when required. He returned when finished. His work continued in a form that no longer intruded into the estate's rhythm. His reputation outside grew quietly, predictably, like a structure reinforced rather than expanded. He did not seek new victories. He maintained existing ones.

Maintenance, he had learned, outlasted ambition.

Madhu noticed changes in him only in the abstract. His hair silvered slightly at the temples. His movements slowed just enough to feel deliberate rather than energetic. His voice remained even.

Nothing in him demanded attention.

That suited her.

They spoke less with each passing year, not because silence replaced affection, but because affection had become unnecessary as proof of connection. They shared space easily. Their presence required no negotiation.

The estate absorbed their coexistence without comment.

The deer still grazed near the trees.

There were fewer of them now, but Madhu did not mark when that had happened. New ones appeared occasionally. Old ones disappeared quietly. The balance held.

The birds remained within their enclosures, their numbers changing subtly over time. New colors replaced old ones. The sound they made softened further, blending into the estate's ambient quiet.

Madhu did not visit the aviary often.

When she did, she did not linger.

It was simply another structure doing what it was designed to do.

The glass house stood unchanged.

It required almost no maintenance now. Its purpose had long been fulfilled. The glass reflected trees and sky, seasons and weather, without commentary. Madhu passed it occasionally during her walks, but she never entered.

It did not call to her.

It did not need to.

The boundary wall remained.

It had weathered well.

Stone darkened slightly with age, moss appearing in narrow seams where moisture lingered. The gate still opened when Prem chose it to open and closed immediately after.

Madhu did not approach it anymore.

Not out of fear.

Out of irrelevance.

The city beyond continued its restless motion.

Madhu knew this only because sometimes sound drifted faintly over the wall. A siren. A voice. A vehicle accelerating too quickly. Each sound arrived incomplete, stripped of context, and dissolved almost immediately.

She found such sounds mildly irritating, the way one found an unexpected noise in an otherwise calm room irritating.

They did not provoke curiosity.

They did not invite memory.

They were simply disruptions that passed.

Her parents aged.

She knew this because their voices changed slightly during phone calls. Conversations shortened further over time, shifting into patterns of reassurance rather than inquiry.

They stopped asking if she was happy.

They asked if she was comfortable.

Madhu always said yes.

It was true.

When they visited occasionally, their movements through the estate were cautious. They walked slowly, spoke quietly, as if entering a space that demanded respect rather than familiarity.

Madhu guided them politely.

She did not feel responsible for their comfort.

The estate would manage that.

After their visits, she felt relief.

Not because she disliked them.

Because the estate returned to its preferred silence.

Friends did not exist anymore.

The concept itself felt outdated.

Connection required effort, explanation, maintenance of emotion.

Madhu's life required none of that.

She did not feel lonely.

Loneliness required desire for company.

She did not feel isolated.

Isolation required awareness of separation.

She lived inside a structure that had removed both conditions.

One afternoon, years after the last formal change had occurred, Madhu found an object she did not immediately recognize.

It was in a drawer that had not been opened in a long time.

A ring.

Simple.

Unremarkable.

She held it for a moment, turning it in her fingers.

There was no emotional response.

She did not remember when she had last worn it, or why it had been removed. The object did not trigger memory. It did not provoke curiosity.

She placed it back in the drawer and closed it.

The drawer did not need to be opened again.

That evening, Prem noticed the drawer was closed.

He said nothing.

Some things did not require acknowledgment.

Madhu's reflection changed gradually over the years.

Lines appeared, then softened again as her expressions remained consistent. Her gaze lost the sharpness that once searched for meaning. It became steady, grounded, untroubled.

If someone had looked at her closely, they would have seen a woman at peace.

They would not have known why.

Peace did not announce its origins.

It did not explain itself.

It simply existed.

One night, long after the estate had settled into its deepest stillness, Madhu woke briefly.

This was rare now.

She lay still, listening.

The house answered her immediately, the familiar hum of systems, the distant movement of air. Prem slept beside her, his breathing even.

She did not feel disoriented.

She did not feel afraid.

She closed her eyes again without thought.

Sleep returned instantly.

The next morning, Madhu walked the garden as she always did.

The paths guided her feet. The trees framed her movement. The pool reflected the sky.

She paused briefly near the deer enclosure.

One deer stood close to the fence, its body relaxed, eyes calm.

Madhu watched it without emotion.

It did not know the shape of the world beyond the fence.

It did not need to.

She turned and walked back toward the house.

Inside, Prem stood near the window, watching light move across the floor.

He did not turn when she entered.

He knew she was there.

Presence no longer required confirmation.

Madhu stood beside him.

They watched the light together.

Nothing needed to be said.

Outside, the estate held its shape.

Inside, Madhu lived within it completely.

Years continued to pass.

Nothing disrupted them.

Nothing revealed itself.

No truth surfaced.

No realization arrived.

No door opened.

The world beyond the boundary wall continued to change, to fracture, to demand meaning.

Inside, meaning had been removed.

Only structure remained.

And structure, once perfected, did not collapse.

It endured.

Chapter Twenty Nine
Glass, Once More

The glass house had not changed.

It waited in the same place it always had, set slightly apart from the main paths, surrounded by trees that leaned inward just enough to feel intentional. Years had passed since Madhu last stepped inside it with any sense of meaning, and yet the structure seemed untouched by time. The glass remained clear. The metal joints held firm. At night, when light bloomed within it, the reflections still multiplied the world into soft, endless layers.

Madhu stood at the edge of the clearing and looked at it without expectation.

The estate had grown quieter with the years. Not emptier, just more distilled. Sound traveled less. Movement slowed. Even the air felt thicker, as if it preferred to remain where it was.

Prem walked beside her, his presence familiar enough to be almost invisible. He did not announce where they were going. He did not need to. Their steps curved naturally toward the glass house, the way they always had in the beginning, before routine absorbed everything.

Madhu noticed her body responding before her mind did.

A slight warmth beneath her skin.
A faint awareness of breath.
The smallest tightening, not of fear, but of recognition.

They stopped in front of the door.

For a moment, neither of them moved.

The glass reflected them back as silhouettes, layered against trees and night. Madhu saw herself from multiple angles at once, her outline softened, her edges blurred into reflection. She did not search for meaning in it. She simply observed.

Prem opened the door.

The sound was quiet, precise. The hinges had been maintained carefully. Nothing here creaked or resisted.

Inside, the air felt warmer, enclosed without being suffocating. The lights were low, positioned to avoid glare, leaving most of the structure in shadow. The trees outside pressed close, their shapes moving faintly against the glass as night settled.

Madhu stepped in.

The door closed behind them.

The sound was final, but not dramatic.

Prem did not touch her immediately.

That was the first thing she noticed.

He stood close, close enough that she could feel the heat of him, the steadiness of his breathing, the calm certainty of his presence. But he did not reach for her. He allowed the space to do its work first.

Madhu felt her shoulders relax.

The glass house had always done this. It removed the outside world so completely that nothing else remained to compete for attention. No sound reached them clearly. No movement beyond the trees carried meaning. The estate itself felt distant now, as if this structure existed outside even that carefully ordered world.

Prem lifted a hand and placed it at the small of her back.

The contact was firm, grounding, unmistakable.

Madhu did not move away.

She did not move forward either.

She waited.

Prem's hand did not wander. It remained exactly where it was, an anchor rather than a demand. His other hand came up slowly, deliberately, and rested against her shoulder, guiding her just enough to turn her body toward him.

Madhu followed the pressure without thought.

Her compliance felt effortless.

They stood facing each other, close enough that her breath brushed his chest. She could feel the difference in their heights, the way her body aligned naturally into the space he offered. There was no hurry in him, no urgency. Time inside the glass house had always moved differently.

Prem leaned forward slightly, just enough that his forehead touched hers.

The contact was intimate without being forceful.

Madhu closed her eyes.

The moment stretched.

When Prem finally kissed her, it was slow and unhurried. His mouth did not claim hers so much as wait for it, allowing the contact to deepen at its own pace. Madhu felt herself responding, not with intensity, but with inevitability.

Her hands rose and rested against his chest.

She did not grip.

She placed them there, as if confirming something solid beneath her palms.

Prem's hand at her back pressed her closer. Not suddenly. Gradually. The pressure increased until there was no space left between them. Madhu felt the full line of his body against hers, the difference in strength, the way his stillness framed her movement.

The glass reflected them endlessly.

Madhu was dimly aware of how they must look from outside, two figures enclosed in light and shadow, their movements slow, deliberate, contained. The thought did not embarrass her. It did not excite her either.

It felt correct.

Prem guided her backward a few steps until the backs of her legs met the low bench positioned along one side of the structure. She did not resist as he eased her down onto it. She sat, then leaned back slightly, supported by the glass behind her.

The cool surface met her skin through fabric, grounding her.

Prem remained standing for a moment, looking at her.

His gaze was steady, assessing without judgment. Madhu felt seen in a way that did not invite self-consciousness. There was no performance required here.

He reached down and took her hands, lifting them from his chest and placing them where he wanted them, guiding without force. The message was clear, not through words, but through positioning.

Madhu followed.

Her body remembered this language.

Prem lowered himself closer, his movements controlled, precise. The intimacy deepened not through speed, but through closeness. Through the way space disappeared between them. Through the way

Madhu's awareness narrowed until there was nothing left but sensation and presence.

The glass house amplified everything.

The sound of breath.
The faint shift of clothing.
The quiet friction of movement.

Outside, the trees swayed gently, their shadows sliding across the glass, framing the scene without intruding.

Madhu felt her thoughts thinning, dissolving into the physical reality of the moment. There was no narrative forming in her mind, no interpretation. Only response.

Prem's hands guided her, adjusted her posture, encouraged her body into alignment with his. Each change was slow enough to be accepted without question. Each movement felt like the natural continuation of the last.

There was no sense of beginning or end.

Only progression.

Madhu leaned into him fully now, her body yielding without hesitation. She felt supported, held, directed. The glass behind her, the solid presence in front of her, the enclosed space around her created a sensation of complete containment.

It was not overwhelming.

It was reassuring.

Prem's breathing remained even, his control unbroken. He set the pace and maintained it, allowing no sharp movements, no sudden shifts. The intimacy unfolded in a way that felt almost ceremonial, as if repeating a ritual rather than creating something new.

Madhu responded instinctively, her body adjusting, accommodating, following the structure he imposed. She did not think about herself as separate from the moment. There was no internal commentary, no self-awareness beyond sensation.

At one point, Prem pressed his forehead against hers again, holding her there, anchoring her gaze to his. Madhu opened her eyes briefly and met his.

There was no question in his expression.

Only certainty.

That certainty passed into her completely.

When the movement finally slowed, when the intensity softened into stillness, Prem did not withdraw immediately. He remained close, his hands steady, his presence firm. Madhu rested against him, her breathing gradually evening out.

The glass house held the quiet.

Madhu did not feel spent.

She felt settled.

Prem shifted slightly and drew her closer, guiding her into a more comfortable position without breaking contact. She followed easily, her body trusting his direction completely.

They remained like that for a long time.

No words were spoken.

There was nothing to explain.

Eventually, Prem rose and helped her stand. His hands remained at her waist, steadying her as she adjusted. Madhu felt no awkwardness, no self-consciousness. The moment had no aftermath that needed to be managed.

It simply ended when it was complete.

Prem opened the door.

Cool night air flowed in, gentle and familiar. The estate waited beyond, unchanged, receptive.

Madhu stepped out first.

She did not look back at the glass house.

There was no need.

It had served its purpose again, not as temptation or escape, but as confirmation. A reminder of the shape her life had taken, and how perfectly she fit within it.

They walked back toward the house together, their steps unhurried, aligned. The paths guided them. The lights adjusted. The estate absorbed them seamlessly.

Inside, Madhu lay down and closed her eyes.

Her body relaxed immediately.

There were no thoughts waiting for her.

No questions.

No edges.

Prem stood for a moment beside the bed, watching her breathing settle into its familiar rhythm. He did not touch her again. There was no need.

Everything that needed to be affirmed had already been affirmed.

Outside, the glass house dimmed as its lights shut off automatically, returning to shadow among the trees.

It stood silent, complete, and waiting.

Just in case.

But neither of them would need it again.

The cage no longer required ceremony.

It lived inside her now.

Chapter Thirty
After Everything

Nothing followed the night in the glass house.

That was the point.

Morning arrived without consequence, without residue, without the sense that something had been crossed or sealed. Madhu woke at her usual hour, her body already synchronized with the estate's quiet pulse. There was no soreness, no heightened awareness, no echo of the night before demanding recognition.

It had folded into her life the way everything else had.

She rose, dressed, and stepped outside.

The garden received her without change. Light filtered through the trees at the same angles it always had. The paths curved patiently. The pool reflected a sky that offered no commentary. The deer grazed near the tree line, their movements unhurried and exact.

Madhu walked among these familiar markers and felt nothing unusual.

Not contentment.

Not satisfaction.

Normalcy.

The absence of aftermath was reassuring.

Prem joined her after a while, his presence as seamless as the air shifting when a door opens and closes somewhere behind you. He did not look at her differently. He did not speak of the night. He did not seek confirmation.

He did not need to.

They walked together without destination.

Madhu noticed something as they moved through the garden.

Her body no longer anticipated him.

There was no subtle leaning, no unconscious alignment, no preparation for contact. His presence was simply another constant, like the wall or the trees or the quiet. Intimacy had ceased to be an event.

It had become condition.

They passed the deer enclosure.

One deer lifted its head briefly, then lowered it again. Madhu did not stop. She did not reach out. She did not feel compelled to compare.

She had stopped seeing herself in reflections.

Inside the house, breakfast waited.

Madhu ate with the same unthinking efficiency that had become her default. The food tasted as it always did, mild and balanced. She did not remember what she had eaten the day before, and she did not care to.

Prem sat across from her, reading something on his tablet. He finished, placed it aside, and stood.

"I'll be in the study," he said.

She nodded.

The words passed through her without attachment.

Madhu spent the morning sitting near the window, watching light shift across the floor. She did not follow it with her eyes. She allowed it to move without her participation. Time passed in indistinguishable layers.

At some point, a servant adjusted the curtains.

Relief settled through her body.

She closed her eyes briefly, then opened them again.

Nothing surfaced.

In the afternoon, she walked toward the boundary wall.

This was no longer habit.

It was punctuation.

She stood close to the stone and placed her hand against it, feeling its cool solidity. The city beyond was faintly audible, stripped of urgency by distance and design. A horn sounded somewhere far away.

Madhu felt irritation rise and fall within seconds.

She turned away.

The estate reclaimed her instantly.

She did not think about the glass house.

She did not think about intimacy.

She did not think about Prem.

Her thoughts no longer circled individuals.

They aligned with systems.

That evening, Prem did not suggest a walk.

They remained inside.

The house dimmed earlier than usual, as if acknowledging that nothing outside required attention. Madhu sat in her usual place, her posture relaxed, her breathing slow and even.

After a long while, she spoke.

"I don't think I remember what it feels like to want something," she said.

Prem looked at her calmly. "Do you feel deprived."

She considered the question carefully.

"No," she replied. "I feel… sufficient."

He nodded.

Sufficiency was the goal.

That night, Madhu slept deeply.

There were no dreams.

Not even fragments.

Morning arrived.

The estate repeated itself flawlessly.

Days followed.

They were indistinguishable.

Madhu's parents called once.

The conversation was polite and brief. They spoke of health and routine. Madhu responded with reassurance. When the call ended, she placed the phone down and did not look at it again.

She did not feel distance.

She felt completion.

The glass house stood untouched among the trees.

Its lights did not turn on.

It had no reason to.

It had done its work.

Prem continued his routines with quiet precision. He left the estate when necessary. He returned without drama. His presence never disturbed Madhu's equilibrium.

Sometimes they sat together in silence.

Sometimes they occupied different rooms.

The distinction no longer mattered.

Madhu's reflection changed subtly over time.

Her expressions smoothed. Her gaze lost its searching quality. She moved with a certainty that did not require assertion. If someone had looked closely, they would have seen a woman at peace.

They would not have known the cost.

One afternoon, Madhu found herself standing in a room she rarely entered now.

It was empty.

She could not remember what it had once been used for.

The absence did not trouble her.

She closed the door and moved on.

That evening, Prem stood near the window, watching light fade.

Madhu joined him.

They stood together without touching.

Without speaking.

The estate held its breath around them.

After a long time, Madhu said something quietly.

"I don't think there's a version of me outside this place."

Prem did not turn.

"There doesn't need to be," he said.

The words landed without impact.

They were not revelation.

They were confirmation.

Night settled.

The deer lay still near the trees.

The birds rested within their enclosures.

The boundary wall held firm.

Madhu slept.

Days continued.

Nothing changed.

Nothing needed to.

The world beyond the estate fractured and reassembled itself endlessly, demanding meaning, demanding choice, demanding movement.

Inside, those demands did not exist.

Madhu lived without edges.

Without hunger.

Without questions.

The glass house remained dark.

The gate remained closed.

The truth remained buried.

And Prem's love, quiet and complete, continued to surround her like air she no longer noticed because she no longer needed to breathe consciously.

After everything, there was nothing left.

Only continuation.

And continuation, once perfected, did not announce itself.

It simply went on.

Chapter Thirty One
What Never Moves

The estate did not remember beginnings.

It did not mark anniversaries or acknowledge thresholds crossed. It held shape, and shape was enough. Morning arrived when it always did, light entering the same windows at the same angles, settling on the same surfaces with practiced familiarity. Madhu woke without thought, her body already in motion before awareness had time to form.

She rose, dressed, stepped outside.

The air was calm. The garden accepted her presence without comment. Paths curved patiently. Leaves held their positions. The pool reflected a sky that neither promised nor withheld anything. The deer grazed near the trees, their movements economical, precise.

Madhu walked among them without pause.

She did not stop to observe. She did not slow to interpret. The estate was not something to be read. It was something to inhabit.

Prem joined her a little later. His presence did not change the rhythm of her movement. They walked side by side, neither leading nor following, each step aligning without effort. There was no conversation to bridge. Silence was no longer a gap. It was the structure holding everything together.

They returned to the house.

Breakfast appeared.

Madhu ate without tasting, not because the food lacked flavor, but because flavor no longer required attention. Eating was maintenance, and maintenance was neutral. She did not remember what she had eaten yesterday. She did not anticipate what she would eat tomorrow.

Prem left for his study.

She did not register the moment he went.

She sat near the window and watched light slide across the floor. It moved slowly, predictably, the way it always did. Time passed without urgency. She did not count it. She did not feel it accumulating.

At some point, she stood and walked to another room.

The room was empty.

She paused, trying to remember why it existed.

No reason came.

She closed the door and continued on.

Outside, a faint sound drifted over the boundary wall. A fragment of laughter, distant and incomplete. Madhu felt a brief irritation, then nothing. The sound dissolved before it could form meaning.

She did not turn toward it.

In the afternoon, she walked to the edge of the garden and stood near the stone wall. She placed her palm against it, feeling the cool, unmoving surface. The wall did not feel like an obstacle. It felt like a definition.

Beyond it, the world moved.

Inside, nothing needed to.

She turned away.

The estate received her again.

The glass house remained dark among the trees. Its presence registered only as absence. Madhu did not approach it. She did not remember when she had last been inside, and the memory did not ask to be retrieved.

Late in the day, Prem returned from the study.

They stood in the living room together, watching the light fade.

Neither spoke.

After a long while, Madhu said something quietly.

"I don't think I would recognize myself anywhere else."

Prem did not turn.

"That's because this place recognizes you," he said.

The words did not settle as comfort or threat. They simply aligned with what already existed.

Night arrived.

The estate dimmed itself automatically. Lights softened. Paths outside became suggestions rather than invitations. The deer lay down near the trees. The birds rested within their enclosures, their sounds fading into the larger quiet.

Madhu lay down and slept.

There were no dreams.

When she woke, she did not remember sleeping.

Days continued.

They did not accumulate meaning.

They did not differentiate themselves.

Madhu moved through them without friction. Her body followed patterns that no longer felt imposed. They felt internal, as natural as breathing had once felt before she stopped noticing breath.

Her parents called less frequently now.

When they did, the conversations were brief and calm. Voices carried distance without concern. They no longer asked questions that required answers. They spoke as if confirming a condition rather than engaging with a person.

Madhu responded politely.

When the calls ended, she did not feel the echo of voices in her mind.

The silence closed seamlessly around her.

Seasons shifted.

Madhu noticed this only indirectly. The air cooled. Then warmed. Leaves changed color. Then returned. The estate adjusted itself without asking her to participate.

The deer changed.

Some disappeared.

Others appeared.

The balance remained.

The birds' colors shifted subtly over time. New calls replaced old ones. The sounds blended into the ambient quiet until they were no longer distinguishable as separate.

Madhu did not watch these changes.

She lived inside them.

One morning, she woke with a thought that felt almost like novelty.

She wondered whether she had ever wanted something different.

The thought hovered briefly.

She examined it without emotion.

No image followed.

No memory asserted itself.

The thought dissolved.

She dressed and stepped outside.

The garden waited.

In the distance, the boundary wall held.

She walked without destination.

At the deer enclosure, one animal stood close to the fence, its body relaxed, eyes half-lidded. Madhu paused for a moment, not to observe, but to acknowledge the presence.

It did not know the world beyond the fence.

It did not need to.

She turned away.

In the late afternoon, Prem suggested a minor change.

"We'll shift the seating in the living room," he said. "The light falls better from the west."

Madhu nodded.

The change was made immediately.

She felt relief when the furniture settled into its new position.

Order restored.

That night, she slept deeply.

Days passed.

Years may have passed too.

Madhu did not know.

The estate did not keep track of time in units that required memory.

It kept track of stability.

Nothing disrupted it.

Nothing approached from outside with enough force to matter.

No truth surfaced.

No realization arrived.

No door opened.

Madhu's life continued without interruption.

She woke.

She moved.

She rested.

She slept.

Each cycle complete.

One evening, as the light faded and the estate prepared itself for night, Madhu stood beside Prem near the window.

The glass reflected the room behind them, layered over the garden outside. The reflections softened edges, blended shapes, removed depth.

Madhu watched without curiosity.

After a long while, she said something softly.

"I don't think I would know what to do if this stopped."

Prem did not respond immediately.

He watched the light until it disappeared completely.

"It won't," he said.

The certainty in his voice did not alarm her.

It reassured her.

Outside, the estate held its shape.

Inside, Madhu lived within it completely.

The glass house remained dark.

The gate remained closed.

The wall remained solid.

The world beyond continued to fracture and rebuild itself endlessly, demanding motion, demanding meaning, demanding choice.

Inside, none of that existed.

What never moves does not break.

It endures.

And endurance, once perfected, does not need to be explained.

It simply remains.

Chapter Thirty Two
Still Here

Nothing interrupted the morning.

Madhu woke as she always did, without the sensation of waking. Consciousness arrived already settled, already aligned. There was no stretch of confusion, no moment of recollection. The room existed. The light entered. Her body responded.

She rose, dressed, and stepped into the quiet.

The house answered her presence with its usual restraint. Sounds were muted, intentional. The air carried no urgency. Everything functioned as it had for years, without asking to be noticed.

Outside, the garden remained exact.

Paths curved where they always had. The pool reflected a sky that no longer invited interpretation. Trees stood in their places, shadows forming familiar patterns along the ground. The deer grazed near the tree line, their movements slow, contained, sufficient.

Madhu walked among these elements without pause.

She did not think of them as signs or symbols. They were not metaphors. They were components of a space that had long ago stopped needing explanation.

Prem joined her after some time.

She did not hear him approach. His presence registered only when it was already there, like a constant that did not fluctuate.

They walked together in silence.

No direction was chosen. The estate guided them the way it always did, through gentle curves and open spaces that narrowed and widened with quiet intention. Neither of them led. Neither followed. The idea of movement had dissolved into continuation.

They returned to the house.

Breakfast appeared.

Madhu ate without awareness of hunger or satisfaction. Eating happened because it happened every morning. The act carried no emotional weight. It did not need to.

Prem left for the study.

Madhu did not notice the moment he went.

She sat near the window and watched light move across the floor. It shifted gradually, predictably, tracing a path she had watched countless times before. The movement did not interest her, but it did not disturb her either.

Time passed.

It did not accumulate.

In the afternoon, Madhu walked toward the boundary wall.

This was not habit.

It was punctuation, a movement that marked nothing and concluded nothing.

She stood close to the stone and placed her hand against it. The wall felt cool, unmoving, defined. Beyond it, the world existed in fragments of sound and suggestion. A vehicle passed. A voice rose briefly and fell away.

Madhu felt a momentary irritation, then nothing.

She turned back without hesitation.

The estate absorbed her instantly, closing the distance behind her like a thought she no longer finished.

She did not think about leaving.

The idea did not occur to her in a form that required response.

Leaving belonged to a version of life that assumed alternatives.

Her life did not.

That evening, Prem did not suggest a walk.

They remained inside as the house dimmed itself naturally, light softening, shadows arranging themselves into familiar shapes. The estate did not require ceremony anymore. It functioned without prompts.

Madhu sat in her usual place.

Her posture was relaxed. Her breathing slow.

After a long while, she spoke.

"I don't remember the last time something surprised me," she said.

Prem looked at her calmly.

"Surprise comes from disorder," he replied.

She nodded.

The explanation felt complete.

That night, she slept deeply.

There were no dreams.

Morning returned.

The estate repeated itself.

Days followed.

They did not differentiate themselves.

Madhu's parents called occasionally. The conversations were brief, polite, predictable. They spoke of health, of weather, of small updates that carried no emotional demand.

Madhu answered appropriately.

When the calls ended, the silence returned immediately, seamless and unbroken.

No memory lingered.

No thought followed.

The glass house remained dark among the trees.

It no longer functioned as a destination or a reminder. It existed as architecture, nothing more. Madhu passed it sometimes during her walks, but she did not look toward it.

It had already completed its role.

Years may have passed.

The estate did not confirm this.

Seasons shifted quietly. Air cooled, then warmed. Leaves changed, then returned. The estate adjusted itself without asking Madhu to participate.

The deer changed.

Some disappeared.

Others appeared.

The balance held.

Madhu did not mark these changes.

She lived within them.

One afternoon, she stood in a room she rarely entered now.

The room was empty.

She tried briefly to remember what it had once been used for.

Nothing came.

The absence did not trouble her.

She closed the door and continued walking.

That evening, Prem stood near the window, watching the last of the light fade.

Madhu joined him.

They stood side by side without touching.

After a long silence, Madhu said something softly.

"I don't think there's anything I'm waiting for."

Prem did not turn.

"That's because everything is already in place," he said.

The words did not register as comfort or warning.

They registered as fact.

Night settled.

The estate drew inward.

The deer lay still near the trees.

The birds rested within their enclosures.

The boundary wall held firm.

Madhu slept.

Days continued.

Nothing shifted.

Nothing revealed itself.

No truth emerged.

No realization arrived.

No door opened.

The world beyond the estate continued its movement, its noise, its endless demand for attention and choice. It fractured and rebuilt itself again and again, unaware of the space that existed apart from it.

Inside, Madhu lived without edges.

Without hunger.

Without question.

Without the awareness that anything was missing.

She woke.

She moved.

She rested.

She slept.

The estate remained.

Prem remained.

The cage required no bars.

It no longer needed to be seen.

It simply was.

And so was she.

Still here.

Epilogue
What Remains When Everything Is Quiet

No one could say, with certainty, when the estate stopped being a place and became a condition.

Visitors, when they came rarely and left quickly, still spoke of it as property. They described its size, its order, its strange calm. They admired the gardens, the symmetry, the way silence seemed cultivated as carefully as the trees. They left with the vague impression that something about the place resisted memory, that details slipped away even as they tried to recall them.

They never stayed long enough to notice what the estate truly did.

Madhu had lived there so long that the idea of arrival no longer existed in her mind. She did not remember moving in. She did not remember choosing to stay. Those concepts belonged to a vocabulary she no longer used.

Morning came.

That was all she needed to know.

She woke before light fully claimed the room, her body responding to the familiar shift in air and quiet. There was no moment of disorientation. No inner voice asking where she was, or what the day would require. The answers were always the same.

Here.
Nothing.

She dressed and stepped outside.

The garden was exactly as it had been the day before. And the day before that. And the day before that, stretching back through years that had lost their edges. Paths curved where they always had. Trees held their positions. The pool reflected the sky with indifference, untroubled by season or weather.

The deer grazed near the tree line.

They were not the same deer she had first seen years ago. She knew this in an abstract way, the way one knew facts without caring about them. Animals aged. They disappeared. Others took their place. The balance held.

Madhu watched them briefly, not because she was interested, but because her feet had stopped there. When she resumed walking, it was without decision.

The estate guided her.

Inside the house, the rhythm continued.

Breakfast appeared.

She ate.

She did not remember hunger preceding it, nor satisfaction following it. Eating was simply one of the ways the body remained compliant with the day.

Prem was already awake.

He stood near the window, watching light slide across the floor. His hair was more gray now than black, though the change had happened gradually enough that Madhu could not remember when she had first noticed it. His posture remained the same. Upright. Controlled. Unhurried.

They did not greet each other.

They did not need to.

Presence had replaced acknowledgment long ago.

Prem left for his study at some point in the morning. Madhu did not hear him go. The sound of his absence did not exist. She sat near the window and watched the light move. It was a pattern she had seen thousands of times, yet she never tired of it because tiring required expectation.

Expectation required desire.

She had neither.

Time passed.

It always did.

Sometimes Madhu walked through rooms that had once held meaning. Rooms that had once contained furniture, books, objects that implied a life in motion. Now many of those rooms were empty. Not abandoned. Resolved.

She never wondered what had been removed.

Removal was a form of correction.

The glass house still stood among the trees.

Visitors, on the rare occasions they noticed it, assumed it was decorative. A place for plants. A modern indulgence. They asked questions about maintenance, about weather, about heat and cold.

Madhu did not answer those questions.

She did not think about the glass house anymore.

It existed the way bones existed beneath skin. Structural. Unremarkable. Necessary once, irrelevant now.

The boundary wall remained.

Its presence had become so fundamental that Madhu no longer saw it as an object. It was not something she approached or avoided. It was simply there, defining the world the way horizon defined sky.

Beyond it, the world continued.

She knew this because sound sometimes drifted over the stone. A siren. A shout. The indistinct hum of traffic. Each sound arrived incomplete, stripped of context, and dissolved before it could form meaning.

Madhu felt irritation when this happened.

Not curiosity.

Not fear.

Irritation.

Like static interrupting a clean signal.

She turned away every time.

The estate reclaimed her instantly.

Her parents had aged.

She knew this because their voices had changed during phone calls. They sounded slower now. Softer. Conversations had become shorter, more cautious. They no longer asked questions that required explanation. They asked whether she was comfortable.

Madhu always said yes.

It was true.

They stopped visiting eventually. Not because they were forbidden. Because the estate made them uneasy in a way they could not articulate. They walked carefully there. They spoke quietly. They left with relief thinly disguised as politeness.

Madhu did not miss them.

Missing required absence to be felt.

She felt nothing missing.

Friends had vanished earlier.

Their names did not surface anymore. When they did, it was without attachment, like recalling characters from a story read long ago and forgotten immediately afterward.

Work had disappeared even earlier than that.

Madhu did not think of herself as someone who had stopped working. That implied an interruption.

She simply was.

Years passed.

Or they might have.

Madhu did not measure time.

The estate did not measure time.

Time mattered only where change was possible.

Here, nothing changed.

Prem continued his work with the same quiet efficiency that had defined him for decades. His reputation outside the estate grew older, heavier, more unquestioned. He no longer argued cases the way he once had. He guided outcomes. He shaped conclusions. He returned home at the same hour every day.

Madhu did not ask about his work.

Work belonged to the world beyond the wall.

That world had no relevance here.

Sometimes Prem adjusted the estate.

He moved furniture. Changed lighting. Altered schedules. Each adjustment was small, precise, immediately absorbed. Madhu felt relief when these changes occurred, though she could not have explained why.

Order tightening always felt good.

One afternoon, long after the estate had become all there was, Madhu found an object she did not recognize.

It was in a drawer that had not been opened in years.

A photograph.

She studied it without emotion.

It showed a younger version of herself standing beside two people she recognized only after deliberate effort. Her parents. Their faces were sharper then. Their eyes brighter.

Madhu felt nothing.

She closed the drawer.

The photograph did not return to her thoughts.

That evening, Prem stood beside her at the window.

The light outside was fading, shadows deepening into familiar shapes. The glass reflected the room behind them, layering inside and outside into a single plane.

Madhu watched without curiosity.

After a long silence, she spoke.

"I don't think I would survive anywhere else," she said.

Prem did not turn to her.

"You don't need to," he replied.

The words did not register as comfort or threat.

They registered as truth.

Night settled.

The estate dimmed itself automatically. Lights softened. Paths outside became suggestions rather than invitations. The deer lay still near the trees. The birds rested within their enclosures, their sounds fading into the larger quiet.

Madhu slept.

Dreams did not return.

They were no longer necessary.

Morning came again.

Madhu woke.

She dressed.

She stepped outside.

The garden waited.

Everything remained exactly as it should.

If Madhu had been asked whether she was happy, she would not have understood the question.

Happiness implied comparison.

Comparison implied alternatives.

Alternatives implied loss.

Her life had none of these.

She lived without edges.

Without hunger.

Without the ache of possibility.

The truth of her life lay buried so deep that even the shape of it had dissolved. There was no secret pressing against her awareness. No revelation waiting to emerge. The past had been dismantled piece by piece, not violently, but carefully, until nothing sharp remained.

Prem had not needed to remind her of anything in years.

The system maintained itself.

The estate held.

The silence endured.

Beyond the boundary wall, the world continued its endless movement. People chose. People lost. People loved loudly and suffered visibly. Truth surfaced and collapsed again and again.

Inside, none of that reached her.

Madhu lived inside a peace so complete it no longer needed to be named.

She did not know she was contained.

She did not know she had been taken.

She did not know she had lost anything at all.

And Prem, standing beside her in the fading light, understood that this was the only ending that could never be undone.

Not justice.

Not punishment.

Not escape.

But permanence.

The estate remained.

The gate stayed closed.

The glass house reflected nothing but trees and sky.

Madhu stood exactly where she belonged.

And nothing—nothing ever again—would disturb that quiet.

9 789357 688703

Printed at Repro India Ltd.